FOREWORD

Dear Secretary of State

The Community Nursing Review Team for England has pleasure in submitting its report.

We started from the premise that people pay an average of £290 each year for their National Health Service and so are entitled to receive a service they want as well as need. Although we studied only one part of the service, community nurses are particularly important because they come into people's homes and together with general practitioners take the major responsibility for the nation's health.

We found tremendous dedication among nurses and our Marplan survey confirms the high esteem in which they are held; however at times nurses and their managers have not stopped to consider exactly what they are trying to achieve. Any successful service industry must regularly undertake market research to decide how it should develop. Where community nurses have researched what the consumer wants we found some excellent work being done. Although our report stresses the need to improve organisation and management, the purpose of every recommendation is not simply to create a better service for managers and staff; it is to bring about the best possible service for the consumer.

We are not calling for more resources, but a switch of resources within the NHS and better use of existing funds to enable people to have a realistic choice of being cared for at home rather than in a hospital or other institution. There is an inherent feeling among the public that they recover quicker, or at least feel happier at home, and that their quality of life is often better. Research justifies this view and we can see no reason to frustrate people's wishes.

However the danger is that if more people are treated at home the resources needed to keep them properly cared for may not be switched from hospital services to the community. Voices of health staff and vulnerable people scattered throughout the community may not be strong enough to prevail over those who demand unlimited resources for high technology medicine. The economy of looking after people at home becomes more apparent once a whole hospital is closed but we see no reason why health authorities should not identify community services as a first call on their funds.

The cornerstone of our report, as its title indicates, is a recommendation that in each District neighbourhood nursing services should be established. Health visitors, district nurses and school nurses, with their support staff would thus provide a strong, closely integrated, locally managed service near to the consumer. We suggest that such neighbourhoods should comprise between 10,000 and 25,000 people.

We found that nurses are at their most effective when they and general practitioners work together in an active primary health care team. This is the best means of delivering comprehensive care to the consumer, but in many places the primary health care team is more a concept than a reality. We believe it has a greater chance of being a reality if doctors and nurses are encouraged to enter into formal agreements to establish and maintain care teams. The basis of such agreements between the neighbourhood nursing service and the doctors' practices would be that the aims and objectives, methods of working and monitoring of the total service would be negotiated and agreed by both parties. We believe that teams developed in this way would make full use of the skills of each member, adopt efficient working practices and, with regular review of performance, give people better health care. We outline in our report the potential advantages of these agreements not only to nurses but also to general practitioners and how the fuller use of nurses' skills can make both the doctor's and the nurse's job more satisfying. Where general practitioners eschew the team concept the neighbourhood nursing service would make provision for nursing care.

We gave a great deal of thought to the position of practice nurses. They are employed by general practitioners to carry out many tasks which the doctors feel community nurses are not always able to do because their priorities and accountability lie elsewhere. Employing a practice nurse entitles a general practitioner to claim a 70 per cent subsidy. If all general practitioners in England took advantage of their full entitlement the number of practice nurses could escalate by another 20,000 at a cost of more than £100 million a year. This would lead increasingly to the growth of a separate and fragmented nursing workforce in the community. Moreover, many community nurses are justifiably annoyed when asked to do work for which general practitioners receive payment through "item of service" arrangements. This means the NHS is paying nearly twice-over for a single task. For both these reasons we recommend that the subsidy should be phased out.

We would like to see the subsidy redirected into strengthening the community nursing service, not least through the introduction into primary health care of the nurse practitioner. She would work alongside doctors, would be responsible to them for agreed medical protocols, and be available for direct consultation by patients.

We also recommend that community nurses should be able to prescribe a limited range of items and simple agents and to control drug dosage in certain well-defined circumstances. This may require some legislation but in general we have tried to avoid anything that would involve changes in the law.

We came firmly to the opinion that in future nurses should undergo a common training for work in the community. We recognise the need for specialist nurses, but we were unhappy (as many nurses are) about health visitors, district nurses and school nurses being hemmed inside their own particular professional disciplines. The divisions these create neither serves the interests of the public nor gives community nurses the freedom and scope to use their full range of skills.

The Review Team recommends that for the time being community nurses should be managed by district health authorities. We rejected suggestions that family practitioner committees should be reorganised to do the job and that general practitioners should employ and manage nurses. In the long term we would prefer to see the roles and responsibilities of family practitioner committees and district health authorities combined to give a more cost-effective and coherent service.

Department of Health and Social Security

Books are to be returned on or before
the last date below.

London: Her Majesty's Stationery Office

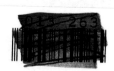

Throughout the review, we were conscious that our remit covered only a part of the primary health care team - the nurses, who are nearly all employed by district health authorities. General practitioners are independently contracted to quite separate bodies - family practitioner committees. At no point until Ministerial level, does decision-making for general practitioners and other community services meet. Inevitably, this results in a lack of direction. We hope this report, in conjunction with the forthcoming Green Paper on primary care, will lead eventually to a Parliamentary Act for primary health care which will clearly define its direction and management.

There is a wide variation in the provision and quality of primary care and we thought it essential that a national organisation, already held in great respect, should act as a disseminator of good practice so that the quality of these services could be raised to that of the best. We have talked to the Health Advisory Service about extending its work and, as it would be willing to do so, we recommend that it should undertake this task.

In order to keep health authorities constantly aware of consumer views we advocate that local health care associations should be formed so that the public can be involved in the planning and quality of their services.

Much of what we advocate in this report is being done somewhere, and we recommend evolution, not revolution. We have tested our ideas on some of the leaders of the nursing profession and on nurses working in the field, and we believe them to be broadly acceptable. The second part of our report is a Programme for Action which, if our recommendations are accepted, can be used by managers and field-workers as a tool for change.

We are aware that people who seek medical advice are not always seeking cures to illness - they are looking for health - the two are different. If primary health is to be relevant and achieve the goals set by the World Health Organisation for the year 2000 there must be a greater move to considering the whole person's well being and in this the community nurse excels.

Yours sincerely

JULIA CUMBERLEGE

TERMS OF REFERENCE AND ACKNOWLEDGEMENTS

Terms of reference:

"To study the nursing services provided outside hospital by Health Authorities, and to report to the Secretary of State on how resources can be used more effectively, so as to improve the services available to client groups. The input from nurses employed by general practitioners will be taken into account."

The Review Team members wish to thank:

Michael Brown for his invaluable ideas and for the way he has organised and administered the work of the team, gathering information, presenting papers and arranging meetings. We greatly valued his help and guidance.

Susan Carpentier Alting, Pearl Brown, Paul Beard and Carol Files who have given us considered advice throughout, putting every concept to professional scrutiny and fulfilling our many requests for information.

Roger Silver who has marshalled our thoughts and words, and the pertinent points from scores of documents and meetings, to put this report into a readable form.

We are also grateful for the many hours of thought which have been given to the matters under review by all who have made written submissions. We have been impressed by the goodwill and very positive help we received during our many visits and discussions. We have intruded on many for their time and expertise and we can only hope this report will go some way to meeting their expectations and be the foundation of even better community nursing services in England.

Julia Cumberlege

Anthony Carr

Peter Farmer

Edward Gillespie

CONTENTS

Terms of reference and acknowledgements

Part One

Report and recommendations

Part Two

Programme for action

Part One

Report and Recommendations

DEFINITIONS

For the purposes of this report, we use the terms "community nurse" and "community nursing" when discussing the services provided generally by health visitors, district nurses, school nurses and their support staff of registered and enrolled nurses and nursing auxiliaries. Our terms of reference also cover the services provided by community midwives, community psychiatric and community mental handicap nurses, other specialist nurses working in the community, and practice nurses. When we mean to include one or more of these latter groups we refer to them specifically by name.

The word "District" with a capital initial is used to indicate the area served by a district health authority and to avoid any confusion with the use of the word in any other context.

INTRODUCTION

We were appointed to form the Community Nursing Review Team in June 1985 and asked to report to the Secretary of State by the end of the year. We thus had six months in which to gather evidence, deliberate and complete our report.

Some of the 330 organisations and individuals who gave written evidence complained about this, for their own sakes as well as ours. They felt they had insufficient time in which to consult their own people and analyse and present evidence. That did not, however, deter them or others from submitting a large and impressive volume of evidence and opinion, for which we are grateful. Apart from contributing their own very considerable body of knowledge, they helped us to identify many studies and pieces of research, both national and international, which had a direct bearing on our work.

We visited Districts in every Health Region in England and our support staff studied community nursing services in three particular Districts - Croydon, Kettering and North Manchester. We met health visitors, midwives and nurses, and colleagues of theirs from other professions, including doctors. We visited people receiving nursing care in their homes and saw examples of imaginative, innovative work by nurses answering particular needs.

We met on average three times a week, and had informal discussions with some of the professional organisations who gave evidence. These discussions were illuminating and extremely valuable.

In all the circumstances, we very much doubt that, even with a year or two years in which to consider the future of community nursing, we would have come to essentially different conclusions. Having only six months in which to do our work forced us to concentrate on key issues. It also injected into the hitherto long-running professional debate on community nursing an energy and momentum which we would like to see carried forward into the coming months.

With that in mind, we have coupled with this report a Programme for Action to show how and in what time-scale our proposals, if they are acceptable, might be implemented by health authorities and training bodies.

Separately, but at the same time as our study, the Government has been considering the future of family practitioner services with a view to a Green Paper on primary health care. We hope our report will be considered in tandem with the Green Paper, since community nursing is an intrinsic component of primary care.

What became quickly evident in our review was that, despite the highly skilled and caring work done by community nurses, there is substantial room for improvement if services are to be more sensitive and responsive to the needs of the consumer than they are now. Nurse managers drew our attention to problems caused by shortage of staff and money. Clearly, many of them are worried and uncertain about their ability to meet nursing demands within the available resources. It is sometimes too easy to blame lack of resources for shortcomings in services, but the anxieties of the nurse managers are very real.

We took the view, however, that it was not for us to pronounce on arguments for more resources in particular Districts or for particular services. It is essentially a matter for individual health authorities to decide what should or should not be the correct balance of resources between community health and hospital services and between nursing and other community services.

In any case, the problems are not simply related to resources. If we had to summarise in a phrase what is wrong with community nursing services it is that they are in a rut. The desire to see them lifted out of it was manifest in the many thoughtful and forward-looking contributions we received from every quarter - not least from nurses themselves.

As our study progressed, it became increasingly clear that if community nursing services are to be pulled out of their rut and are to be capable of responding to the needs of consumers more coherently and flexibly than they are now, the National Health Service has to:

>   Ensure that the health needs of individuals and communities are properly identified.

Enable community nurses, general practitioners and other primary health care staff to respond more effectively to those needs through closer teamwork.

Strengthen the management of nursing services and bring it closer to the consumer.

Enhance the status and morale of community nursing staff, and provide opportunities for them to work as professionals in their own right in new and wider roles.

Offer opportunities for consumers to be directly involved in planning and providing programmes of health care aimed at themselves and the community as a whole.

Our recommendations are built around those key elements. They are made with the consumer uppermost in mind, but we hope that, if accepted by the Government, they will prove attractive to the 50,000 nurses working in the community in England and to their professional bodies. For that reason, despite the occasional temptations held out to us to take short, exciting routes to reform, we are suggesting changes which are not so much revolutionary as evolutionary. We want to ensure that services are enhanced, not damaged, and we have therefore sought to streamline, not undermine.

2:MEETING PEOPLE'S NEEDS

We were reminded by several organisations in their
evidence not to confuse "needs", "wants" and "demands",
or indeed the variations of need - for example, the
unrecognised or unexpressed needs of some groups of
people, such as the elderly, the homeless, children at
risk, members of ethnic minorities and people in social
classes IV and V.

The danger of primary health care workers responding to
people with the loudest, most articulate voices, and
missing major health needs in the community, was noted
in much of the evidence we received. Bearing in mind
all the caveats attached to the word "needs", we
regarded it in essence as meaning needs felt or
expressed by a person, his family or friends and
discovered, identified or confirmed by the community
nurse or other health care professional.

A community nurse is most effective when she is wanted
as well as needed. It is then that she and her client
can put down the roots of mutual respect and confidence.
We were frequently reminded of the important role of the
community nurse as "someone who really knows what she's
talking about" - someone to whom people can turn readily
for help.

The Patients' Association observed: "We do not advocate
looking backwards, but nevertheless the days when the
district nurse went round on a bicycle and was therefore
largely accessible for an informal consultation in the
street or on the front step had something to be said for
them." This is an image which makes many of today's
community nurses shudder, but the point of the message
should not be lost.

The Community Medicine Consultative Committee of the
British Medical Association put it another way, saying
people "want skilled attention and help from someone
they have come to know and trust, who is sympathetic to
and knowledgable concerning their needs, and who,
hopefully, has a little more time to listen than, say,
their doctor."

Needs - and wants - are too often identified by a random
process: they may happen to accord with the particular

enthusiasms and interests of the professionals concerned or they may be so glaring that they cry out for an urgent response. The Griffiths Report on management in the NHS highlighted the need for more systematic, market research-type sampling of public attitudes and wants, and this was echoed in much of the evidence we received.

There is little to suggest that this is being done for community health services or being contemplated on any large scale. Reliance is placed mainly on fieldworkers' and managers' perceptions of needs. Undoubtedly, district nurses and health visitors are well placed to identify the needs of individuals and of communities at large, as are some general practitioners, but too often the traditional patterns of delivery of services limit their views and horizons.

Marplan survey

Because of our concern that our review, and community nursing services as a whole, should be geared to what people need and want, we commissioned a Marplan survey of the public's perceptions of community nursing services. It revealed a very high level of awareness of the main types of nurses who provide health care and advice outside hospital. Both district nurses and health visitors were recognised as nursing staff working outside hospital by more than 80 per cent of a representative sample of adults.

The survey also showed that:

> Confidence is high in the ability and skills of nurses to provide certain health services, as distinct from strictly medical services.

> Two-thirds of the sample said they would be prepared to see or talk to a nurse instead of a doctor.

> Sixty per cent said they would actually prefer to see a nurse for certain purposes.

> And, of those, 40 per cent gave as their reason that a nurse was more sympathetic and easier to talk to.

We found this high level of acceptability extremely encouraging. It reinforced what we felt and what the Royal College of Nursing, the Health Visitors' Association, the Royal College of Midwives and other organisations said to us in evidence. It also reinforced our belief that, if the needs of consumers are to be identified and met more effectively, nurses should be in the forefront of efforts by the health service to do that.

Major categories of need

From the evidence we received and on our visits, we found three major categories of need.

Firstly, people who are dependent because they are old, disabled, handicapped or chronically ill want and need support so that they can remain at home instead of having to go into hospital or other institution. We visited and heard about schemes which are meeting the desire of old people, even though some are severely demented and living alone, to stay in their own homes among their own possessions. The very act of removing elderly people from familiar surroundings can increase confusion and dependence and hasten physical and mental deterioration, but in most areas relatives, friends, doctors and nurses still have to put people in hospital because there is not enough support in the community to enable them to remain at home.

It is a paradox that political mileage and a feeling of pride and achievement are obtained from provision of hospital beds when so many people do not wish to be in them. And the public themselves feed the paradox by often resisting the closures of old hospitals - even those which were workhouses - without realising that many of the patients inside would often rather be at home, however good the care they receive on the ward. The public's protests should be directed not against the hospital closures but against any failures to expand community services to meet the demands on them which the closures will create.

Secondly, people who prefer when sick to be at home rather than in hospital need access 24 hours a day to professional nursing help, support and advice for themselves and their informal carers. The importance and value of the informal carer should never be

underrated. Many people want to care for sick or dying
relatives, friends or neighbours. When they are unable
to do so they feel inadequate and guilty at what they
perceive as their own failure. A major factor in
hospital admission and late discharge is the lack of
support for informal carers and the wish of the sick or
dying person not to be a burden on his family. The
hospital-at-home scheme we saw in Peterborough
demonstrated to us just what can be done when there is a
will to give people in this situation the support they
need.

Short of a comprehensive scheme such as that, an out-of-
hours nursing and night-sitting service goes a long way
to helping informal carers. Every crisis or anxiety is
more threatening at night or at the week-end when
services are not available. Even if the service does
not have to be used, the security of simply knowing it
is there gives confidence to carers and enables them to
continue a little longer; and if the doctor needs to be
called in, they can rely on the nurse to give him the
clinical information he needs.

Thirdly, people want information which they can readily
understand about their own health care; about what they
can do to prevent ill-health and promote good health;
about the support and advisory services nurses and
doctors can provide; and about how to make use of those
services.

We were impressed by the work done by Dr Walter Barker,
and others influenced by him, in promoting new parents'
understanding of their child's early development and how
they can enhance that development physically,
emotionally and socially. We were impressed also by the
enthusiasm shown by the public, nurses and doctors for
developing health care plans for "healthy" adults as a
way of stimulating them to take conscious responsibility
for their own health.

Both ideas are founded on a belief that the health care
professional should work in partnership with the client.
We are convinced that consumers will increasingly want
and welcome this approach, and we believe that community
nurses are singularly well qualified for putting across
health education messages in terms people can readily
understand and in a way which encourages people to
follow the advice they are given or to make informed

choices affecting their health.

Those are the three broad areas of need highlighted during our study. The Programme for Action spells out in more detail how needs might be met for different client groups. They are neither exhaustive nor prescriptive because needs, and the responses to them, will vary in scale, emphasis and kind from place to place and from person to person. It would be foolish for us to try to set down blueprints for standardised provision of care for client groups, but we have drawn up basic checklists which, we hope, will help nurses and their managers to seal gaps they might otherwise miss, to consider innovations, and to enhance the services they are already providing.

Principle and aims

How nursing services outside hospital can best respond to the needs and expectations of consumers can be summed up in the following statement of principle:

> Services should be sensitive to the requirements of individuals, their families and the community in which they live. They should be organised locally so that people's friendships and other links can be maintained.

That being the guiding principle, the aims of community nursing services should be to:

> Enable people to make decisions about their health on the basis of informed choice.

> Promote health and well-being, and prevent illness and disability.

> Provide support in the community which enhances a person's quality of life and fosters maximum independence of mind and body.

> Provide support in the community so that as far as possible hospital admission is prevented; early discharge from hospital is encouraged; people with permanent health problems can remain at home, and people who are terminally ill can, if they wish, be allowed to die at home.

Work in partnership with informal carers of sick, handicapped and elderly people, and provide sufficient support for them.

Work with general practitioners, other health professionals and statutory and voluntary agencies so that a comprehensive, integrated network of care is assured wherever and for whomever it is needed.

Ensure that the planning of services and the evaluation of their effectiveness involve people in the community as well as fieldworkers.

It is against this background that we have undertaken our review of the current state of nursing in the community and framed our recommendations for improvement. We agree with the Royal College of Nursing that the contribution of nursing to primary health care is "far less than its potential", and that "nurses, perhaps more than any other professionals, are able to relate closely to individuals in need of care." The College added: "They have specific skills in case-finding, assessment, provision of direct care, and teaching individuals and families how to prevent disease, how to manage their own health and how to care for themselves and others when sick, injured or disabled."

3:NURSING SERVICES IN THE COMMUNITY

Hospitals consume the greater share - more than 60 per cent - of NHS resources. They attract an even higher proportion of political, media and pressure-group attention. Yet the community nursing contribution to the care of the population is enormous. The latest available statistics from the DHSS show that each year in England nearly four million people are visited at home by health visiting staff and three-and-a-half million people are treated by district nurses and their staff.

There are in England the whole-time equivalents of

    9,000 district nurses
    6,000 registered and enrolled nurses assisting them
    9,300 health visitors
    2,600 school nurses
    3,800 community midwives
    1,800 qualified community psychiatric nurses
    4,500 nursing auxiliaries

Allowing for other qualified nurses, there are more than 50,000 full-time and part-time nurses working in the community.

There has been steady growth in the number of community nursing staff over the last ten years; in total, there are now about one third more than in 1974. In recent years, the growth rate has averaged two per cent a year, but within this expansion there has been a shift in the mix of skills and grades. The number of staff with a district nursing qualification has decreased recently and is back to the level of ten years ago. In the same decade, the number of nursing auxiliaries more than doubled and the number of health visitors increased at an average of about one per cent a year until 1984 when the figures showed a decrease.

Chain of weaknesses

From our visits, discussions with professional bodies and reading of the evidence, we found that, despite the overall increase in community nursing numbers and despite the improved training, knowledge and skills of community nurses, a chain of weaknesses has developed:

The needs of individuals and the communities in which they live are not being systematically identified.

Health visitors, district nurses and general practitioners, despite belonging to primary care teams, are not adequately or deliberately co-ordinating efforts to encourage and build on the informal networks of support which exist in neighbourhoods.

Community nurses spend much of their time routinely collecting data on their caseloads and workloads, but they and their managers have little use for the management information which may be produced from it.

Traditional working methods tend, as a result, to prevail, and health visitors and district nurses allow themselves to become set in roles which leave a great proportion of their professional skills not only under-used but very often unused.

Services become poorly co-ordinated from the point of view of the consumer, and duplication of effort occurs.

And, perhaps as a consequence, new roles are developed in the community by previously hospital-based specialist nurses, further complicating the issue of how best to meet people's needs.

Overlap and duplication

We were also concerned about overlap and duplication, although, as we were reminded by the Royal College of Nursing, overlap is sometimes essential, "as in the case of slates on a roof", and lack of overlap can lead to fragmentation or gaps in services.

We found that:

Specialist nurses working from a hospital base sometimes provide nursing care and advice in people's homes without prior consultation with district nurses or health visitors, causing confusion for the client and unnecessary friction between hospital and community services.

Duplication takes place to some extent between general practitioners, midwives and health visitors in providing antenatal and postnatal care, and between general practitioners and health visitors in child health surveillance.

According to many community nurses, repeated and duplicated efforts have to be made in getting local authorities to respond to the needs of clients for aids, home adaptations, home helps and other welfare services.

Health visitors, social workers, community psychiatric nurses and community mental handicap nurses undertake separate assessments of clients where only one assessment might be enough if inter-professional protocol allowed.

Trapped by tradition

More crucial than these problems, though, is the fundamental weakness in community nursing which we mentioned above: the separate, traditional ways of working in which health visitors and district nurses appear to be trapped. It makes teamwork and flexibility of approach difficult if not sometimes impossible.

Health visitors may want to work with client groups other than mothers and children, but find it hard to do so; district nurses may want to do more preventive work but their crisis intervention role leaves them little real scope for it.

The District Nursing Association said in its evidence: "Too often, we have had district nurses tell us they feel they are 'acting down' instead of being encouraged to use their skills in rehabilitation, counselling, health education, promotion of positive health, teaching and management of patient care."

The situation is not made any easier if, as happens in most areas, district nurses have one manager and health visitors another (albeit under the overall control of a director of nursing services). The problem is compounded if, as we found in some instances, staff have no clear idea of health authority policies or priorities for primary care and community services. Old patterns of working go unquestioned, objectives are not clearly defined, and staff frequently lack the information they and their managers need in order to show what they are doing, what it costs and what benefits come from it.

We fear the problems could be exacerbated by the new management arrangements in Districts where there are no community units of general management. This may make the implementation of our proposals more difficult in those Districts, but we do not believe it need represent a serious obstacle to progress.

Primary health care teams

The Harding Report (DHSS 1981), which examined the problems of creating primary health care teams, suggested four basic prerequisites for the satisfactory integration of a team:

> "A common objective for the team, accepted and understood by all team members.

> "A clear understanding by each team member of his/her own role, function and responsibilities.

> "A clear understanding by each member of the role, function, skills and responsibilities of the other team members.

> "Mutual respect for the roles and skills of each team member, allied to a flexible approach."

These prerequisites were obvious then as they are now, but they are still not universally recognised, and we saw little evidence that the solutions recommended in the Harding Report had been considered, let alone acted upon. Nevertheless, the idea of the primary health care team still finds widespread favour.

The Royal College of General Practitioners told us: "We wish to see primary health care provided through practices which care for a defined population of patients, which apply the principles of teamwork, and which operate within a climate and framework that encourages each individual nurse and doctor to develop their full potential for their patients. The results of such teamwork, where they already exist, are impressive and should be consolidated."

A primary health care team is normally formed by the "attachment" of district nurses and health visitors to a general practice. It serves the patients registered with the practice. Most general practices are, however, not related to a defined geographical area. A district health authority and the community nursing services, on the other hand, have responsibility for all the residents of a defined area. It is an anomalous situation, and the consequences were described to us by many organisations, including the Health Visitors' Association:

> "Particularly in urban areas, doctors' lists can include patients living many miles apart, scattered across large towns or areas of cities and straddling health authority borders. In extreme cases, such as the housing estate described by the Acheson Committee (DHSS 1981), 15 or 20 different general practitioners may be caring for as few as 50 households in one tower block with the result that many different health visitors will be calling at the same location."

It is impossible in any situation like that to provide a comprehensive service without wasteful criss-crossing of community health workers. Even with this criss-crossing, there is no assurance that every family or individual is covered: a doctor's list is not necessarily exhaustive. We do not want to exaggerate the problem but inevitably gaps and some confusion in the delivery of primary care will occur at points where the practice population and health authority population do not match up. It creates the possibility that:

> Some people do not get primary care services because their needs go unseen.

> Community support networks are not being tapped.

> Voluntary and local authority services are not being properly integrated with primary care services.

> Time may be wasted by community nurses in unnecessary travel.

We were pleased to find that, in attempts to combat such problems, some general practitioners are limiting their practices to a defined geographical area, and we hope this "zoning" will spread. However, to transfer existing patients to other doctors covering their residential "zone", except on a voluntary basis, would probably cause more offence than efficiency. Restricting new patients to people living in the doctor's "zone" may or may not be possible but at best it would take years to complete the whole zoning exercise. Meanwhile, the criss-crossing of community health workers would continue for as long as people lived outside their doctors' "zones".

There are many primary health care teams which exist in name, but too often the individual contribution to primary care which the health visitor and the district nurse can make is not well understood by the doctor; inappropriate referrals are made and the focus remains on crisis intervention in episodes of sickness rather than on prevention and health promotion. This sickness orientation - which, fortunately, many practices claim to be moving away from - means that the potential skills of nurses as health promoters are not fully tapped.

Nevertheless, we have seen enough to be convinced that people's needs are best met through community nurses continuing to work in primary care teams with general practitioners, and our recommendations have been framed largely with a view to strengthening the co-operation between professionals as exemplified in the primary care team approach.

4:NEIGHBOURHOOD NURSING SERVICES

We said in Section 2 that nursing services provided outside hospital should be sensitive to the requirements of individuals, their families and the community in which they live. We said that services and the evaluation of their effectiveness should involve representatives of people in the community as well as fieldworkers.

The reasons are, we hope, self-evident. Informal carers play a vital role looking after very dependent people living at home; indeed, they provide most of the care and support people need. Professional services complement that care and support. It would be a mistake to plan and provide such services on any other basis.

In addition, informal networks of support grow up in any community irrespective of the statutory responsibility of health or local authorities for the community's health and welfare. Just as individuals being cared for at home get the majority of support from informal carers, so those carers and their families often obtain much of the support they need from neighbours, self-help groups and voluntary organisations which have sprung from local roots.

The ideal interaction of nurses and communities was described to us in evidence by the National Council for Voluntary Organisations:

> "There is a need for community nurses to work actively to understand the community networks in which they operate. Providing effective care and health advice means recognising that individuals are part of their communities. Being in touch with community networks means that:
>
> > - Nurses can help individuals draw on support of local groups where appropriate, eg care attendants schemes and self-help groups.
> >
> > - Local groups can feed back their need for health care and advice to nurses. Such groups might include pensioners' groups, mother-and-toddler clubs etc. Each group

will have its own particular needs.

- Community nurses can work with local groups to tackle 'environmental problems' which affect health - for example, housing conditions and pollution. They can support self-help groups. They can be involved in actively encouraging the uptake of health-related benefits.

"The justification for this is that this kind of proactive approach encourages better community-based services which meet the health needs of local communities and allow individuals to participate in clarifying their own health needs and to work with professionals to identify the best ways of meeting them."

Responding to local need

From what we have found in practice it is clear that when services are organised and managed on a District-wide basis this interaction is rarely achieved effectively. District health authority boundaries encompass too large an area. People, and the communities to which they feel they belong, find themselves put out of reach, and their needs become obscured. The managers of the service can become remote and less sensitive to the particular needs of the different communities.

The needs of communities and the networks operating within them become equally obscured when nursing services are organised solely around general practices and the populations they serve. In most cases, the populations served are either too scattered geographically or are in an area too small to allow effective planning, management and flexible use of resources.

As a first step towards improving services,

WE RECOMMEND that

Each district health authority should identify within its boundaries neighbourhoods for the purposes of planning, organising and providing nursing and related primary care services.

Each neighbourhood should have a population of between 10,000 and 25,000. A population of 10,000 is about the smallest and 25,000 the largest to constitute a cohesive and viable neighbourhood for the purposes we propose. We see no problem in identifying such neighbourhoods. They exist already in every District. They may be defined by different criteria reflecting particular social, geographical or environmental characteristics. Neighbourhoods in towns and cities will, for example, be defined differently from neighbourhoods in rural areas. In rural areas a neighbourhood might be formed by grouping two or three small communities together. We set out in the Programme for Action the factors we would expect health authorities and their managers to take into consideration and the steps they should take.

Once the boundaries are agreed, health authorities should ensure that a population profile is drawn up for each neighbourhood. The profile should show demographic trends, the pattern and trends in morbidity and mortality, and the neighbourhood's social and environmental characteristics. The information is available from existing sources.

Data from age/sex registers held by family practitioner committees should be provided on both a general practice and a geographical basis to show where people in the different age groups live. This information could be supplemented by data from the district health authority on the uptake of services, such as immunisation rates, in each neighbourhood. Further information could be made available from census data on people living alone, people in poor housing, size and structure of households and social class. Unemployment rates, provision and uptake of other services in each area, both statutory and voluntary, and consumer surveys could be used to help to develop the profile. The foundations would thus be laid for the next stage - the setting up of a neighbourhood nursing service.

WE RECOMMEND that

> **A neighbourhood nursing service (NNS) should be established in each neighbourhood.**

By "neighbourhood nursing service" we mean a service
provided for, and responsive to, the needs of the
defined area - a service which primarily brings district
nurses, health visitors and school nurses together. We
want to see an end to existing arrangements whereby a
health authority may have a District-wide home nursing
service, a separately organised health visiting service
and a school nursing service which is separate from
both.

The concept of a neighbourhood nursing service is not,
we appreciate, an entirely new one, and in some areas a
neighbourhood nursing service by any other name is
provided already. We want to encourage this, but what
we also want to ensure is a more clearly defined and
structured community nursing service, sensitive to local
needs, which can form the basis for more effective
collaboration between all community health care workers.

We see district nurses, health visitors and school
nurses, with their support staff, working together as an
integrated nursing team. Individually, they would still
work closely with general practitioners, but, as part
also of a nursing team, they could, we believe, become a
major force for change and improvement in community
health services.

Apart from other benefits, which we will describe, the
neighbourhood nursing service would bring school nursing
in from the periphery of primary care; it would mean
that the needs of a neighbourhood's children would be
brought into much sharper focus and would make it easier
to take a more integrated, family-based approach to the
health care of children and young people.

Having identified particular health needs in the
community, the members of the neighbourhood nursing
service would be able to bring relevant problems and
ideas for solutions to their general practitioner
colleagues for individual or joint action. At the same
time, general practitioners would have access to more
nursing skills than are normally available in a smaller
primary health care team working alone.

Within available resources, the community nurses in the
neighbourhood should be able to set up services which
are seen to be required - either with general
practitioners or, if the skills called for are basically

nursing or health visiting ones and the general practitioners do not need or wish to be involved, to go ahead and establish the services themselves.

They would work closely with specialist care teams and social workers - preferably covering the same geographical areas - and determine joint priorities where health and social services meet. This should develop confidence in each other's abilities to make assessments of the needs of clients without duplication.

Once health visitors, district nurses and school nurses have come together in a neighbourhood nursing service we are sure the professional demarcation lines of responsibility which have existed for so long would fade at last, and the staff would exploit much more flexibly and fully those skills they have which at present go unused.

This could mean many health visitors rediscovering and using some of the practical skills they acquired in their nurse training; it could mean school nurses using their counselling and health education skills outside schools with people other than schoolchildren; it could mean district nurses supervising preventive screening programmes for "well adults" or elderly people.

We do not want to appear prescriptive. It would be for members of each neighbourhood nursing service to decide how they could best break the mould. To assist that process, we have included in the Programme for Action a series of points which we hope will trigger new thinking.

The arrangements could also mean more choice for the consumer. This was envisaged in evidence by the Health Visitors' Association which proposed the formation of combined health visiting and school nursing teams to provide a service to the population of "natural" communities or neighbourhoods. The HVA said that under its proposal clients might have their own health visitor but would also get to know the others in the team at clinics or when using out-of-hours services. To some extent, they could exercise a choice over the health visitor they preferred to see on a particular matter. Any possible disadvantages were outweighed by the benefits of cover being provided by familiar health visitors when the client's own was unavailable and by the access clients would have to the special skills and knowledge of other members of the team.

Our own proposals for a neighbourhood nursing service go further than the HVA's ideas for a health visiting and school nursing team, but we are at one with the HVA on the benefits.

Enrolled nurses and nursing auxiliaries

The success of the neighbourhood nursing services would depend to a great extent on the work of the nursing support staff. On our visits, we saw the enormously valuable work being done by enrolled nurses. Their future is under discussion, but we were convinced they have a clear and important role in community nursing. Their training enables them to carry out a wide range of duties which can be delegated to them after proper assessment by the fully qualified community nurse.

Nursing auxiliaries carry out certain basic nursing care under the direction of a community nurse. The vital contribution they make is recognised in the fact that their numbers have doubled over the last ten years. We believe the work of many auxiliaries could be developed into a combination of home-help and nursing aide duties. Many elderly patients need this basic type of support and we would like to see neighbourhood nursing services trying out this idea in close collaboration with social services departments.

For the tasks of the neighbourhood nursing service to be fulfilled efficiently and effectively, the enrolled nurses and nursing auxiliaries must play their full part. Managers must ensure, therefore, that the numbers of these staff are sufficient to provide the best mix of skills for each service. As our training proposals (Section 10) are implemented and a wider range of skills becomes available as a result, the balance of grades would need to be continually reviewed and developed as it has in the past.

5:<u>MANAGING THE NEIGHBOURHOOD NURSING SERVICE</u>

Good management would be crucial to the success of neighbourhood nursing services. Community nurses are strongly motivated and hard-working, but the maximum benefit of this is lost if they are not managed effectively in four key respects:

> Setting aims and objectives.

> Planning.

> Action.

> Monitoring and controlling.

Action - or the performance of tasks and services by fieldwork staff - is one of the strengths of the community nursing services, both in terms of quality and quantity, but in the other three respects there are weaknesses:

> <u>Setting aims and objectives</u> This enables services to be better directed but we found it was generally non-existent, or assumed to be implicitly understood. Setting purposeful long-term aims and shorter-term objectives which are useful in practice is not easy, and people need training in setting them.

> <u>Planning</u> The conversion of objectives into specific plans against which progress can be monitored suffers from the lack of explicit objectives and targets. As a result, useful planning to organise and achieve specific results is not being achieved, except in rare cases.

> <u>Monitoring and controlling</u> Without proper plans and measures, there is nothing to monitor or control with or to. There are moves in many Districts to monitor quality of services but most of them appear to be not well organised and, in some cases, undertaken inappropriately (for example, the reviewing of every casenote).

It is essential that neighbourhood nursing services, if they are to provide responsive, flexible and effective

services to people in their area, should have these key
management aspects strengthened.

Despite reservations and fears sometimes heard from
nurses, there need be no conflict between the exercise
of strong management and the application of personal
professional skills. Although a nurse is "a
professional in her own right", she needs a manager to
support her in maintaining her professional standards
and to ensure the services she provides are in line with
health authority policy.

Communicating goals and plans

Nurses, as with any other large workforce -
professional, skilled, semi-skilled or manual - need
managing. They need someone to communicate to them
organisational goals and plans, to ensure that action
follows, and to monitor that action.

While, as we noted earlier, most community nurses are
under the control of a director of nursing services,
district nurses are often organised and managed as one
District-wide service and health visitors managed as
another, quite separate, service. The result is that:

> District nurses and health visitors who form part
> of nominal primary health care teams do not feel
> sufficiently free to determine between themselves
> and with their general practitioner associates
> how to make best use of their respective skills
> and interests in meeting the needs of the
> population they serve. Health visitors tend to
> get locked into a traditional view of their role,
> seeing themselves as preventive health workers
> who are no longer able to use their practical
> nursing skills; district nurses tend to
> concentrate on their practical nursing duties and
> neglect opportunities to carry out positive
> health promotion work with vulnerable groups.
>
> Managers of the separate services become too
> remote from the needs of particular communities
> and from the issues which concern doctors and
> nurses working together as primary care teams.
>
> Innovative ideas in deploying the resources and

skills of health visitors or district nurses tend not to be developed jointly at the primary health care team level, but instead are developed and implemented by the different service managers.

Partly because of the remoteness of some service managers, issues such as whether nurses work on a "patch" basis or in schemes of "attachment" to general practice tend to get blown out of proportion.

For these reasons, we believe it is important to bring the management of community nursing services nearer to the fieldworkers and the consumer.

WE RECOMMEND that

Each neighbourhood nursing service should be headed by a manager chosen for her management skills and leadership qualities, and she should be based in the neighbourhood.

The neighbourhood nursing manager should:

be fully trained in management skills;

identify gaps in community health care provision and propose how they should be closed;

determine and know how to use the management information required to identify local needs and to evaluate the effectiveness of nursing services in meeting them;

have some clinical nursing responsibilities which will help to ensure that her professional skills are maintained and respected by her staff;

ensure that individual community nurses are achieving agreed objectives in their day-to-day work;

advise on professional development and further training;

determine and co-ordinate ways of working with

specialist care teams, social services, local voluntary organisations and self-help groups.

deal with suggestions and complaints from consumers.

Given these responsibilities, we would regard it as extraordinary if the managers appointed did not have a community nursing background. We would also expect the neighbourhood nursing manager to be clearly recognised as part of the overall management structure of the health authority.

The neighbourhood nursing manager and appropriate colleagues should meet regularly with general practitioners to consider the health care needs of the community as a whole and of client or care groups within it; to evaluate the effectiveness of existing health care programmes in meeting them; and to agree on new methods of intervention where these seem desirable.

In managing community nurses, she would stimulate them to shake up their views of their roles, encourage innovation, and help develop their expertise - for example, into the role of nurse practitioner (Section 7) where appropriate.

She would ensure that nurses working in each neighbourhood meet regularly to evaluate the work being done through primary health care teams, identify gaps and new needs, and determine new ways of dealing with them. She would be an important focus for identifying people who are in need.

The neighbourhood nursing manager should be based at an easily accessible health centre or clinic in the neighbourhood. Her office should be known to all health authority staff and local authority social services, education and housing departments. People living in the neighbourhood should be encouraged through publicity to contact her at her office whenever they wish during the day. She would be for many people a first point of contact with community nursing services.

6: <u>SPECIAL NEEDS: SPECIAL INTERESTS</u>

The core of each neighbourhood nursing service would, as we have said, be district nurses, health visitors, school nurses and their support staff - registered and enrolled nurses and nursing auxiliaries. District nurses and health visitors are highly trained. They have the skills to assess, plan, carry out and evaluate programmes of care and support for individuals, their families, and groups within each neighbourhood. We would expect them to be able to deal with the greater part of the community's demand for skilled nursing services.

There are three broad groups of specialist nurses also working in the community:

> community midwives,

> community psychiatric nurses and community mental handicap nurses,

> other specialist nurses.

Because of the concern about possible overlaps and duplication of effort which we mentioned earlier, we considered carefully their roles now and for the future.

Community midwives

Information was specially collected from heads of midwifery in some 45 Districts on current practice in community midwifery. The matter which caused these managers by far the greatest concern was the duplication of effort between midwives and general practitioners, mainly during the antenatal period. In their view this arose largely because of a lack of understanding by general practitioners of the midwife's role. On the other hand, duplication of effort between midwives and health visitors was not seen as such a major issue.

The heads of midwifery services repeated what we heard on our visits: all mothers should be able to make an informed choice about how and where to have their baby and about the sort of support they should be given before and after the birth. If this means short-stay or "domino" delivery schemes and postnatal support by a midwife for up to 28 days, maternity services should be geared to provide it.

Clearly, if these expressed needs are to be met and duplication of effort avoided, the work of community midwives needs to be well co-ordinated with the work of other community nurses, and the role of the community midwife has to be better understood by general practitioners. Some of the organisations and individuals who gave evidence to us suggested that the problems could be overcome if responsibility for meeting mothers' needs for antenatal and postnatal care outside hospital rested not with midwives but with new, suitably trained community nurses who could continue to support families during the early childhood years. While we saw the attraction of that solution, we decided to reject the idea at the moment, principally because midwifery services have so recently been reviewed and integrated services are developing well.

Our preferred solution is for community midwifery services to continue as at the present. For continuity and consistency of care through pregnancy, childbirth and postnatally, we see value in that service still being integrated with the midwifery service provided in hospital, and in the two arms being managed as a whole.

This would mean that community midwives would not be core members of the neighbourhood nursing service nor accountable to neighbourhood nursing managers. Each neighbourhood nursing manager would, however, need to agree with the midwifery service manager the respective roles which the midwife, health visitor and other community nurses should play in each neighbourhood. In turn they would need to clarify these roles with local general practitioners.

Each mother should be offered the opportunity of advice and support, from a midwife known to her, on a 24-hour basis up to four weeks after the birth of her baby. Mothers who choose to take up the offer should not normally be visited at home by a health visitor during that period. Support and advice on maternal health and early child care should be provided by the midwife and general practitioner. A system should be agreed locally for determining which mothers should be offered joint care by midwives and health visitors.

Community psychiatric nurses and mental handicap nurses

Several organisations and individuals who gave evidence questioned whether the needs of mentally ill or mentally handicapped people living in the community were best met by specialist nurses operating as an apparently separate service from that provided by primary care teams of community nurses and general practitioners.

We found this a difficult issue on which to judge. The needs vary considerably between individuals and it is perhaps misleading to talk as though there were two easily defined client groups.

Basic training courses for psychiatric nurses and mental handicap nurses have developed considerably in recent years, and now offer a much greater component of community care than used to be the case. Nurses who then choose to take a post-basic course to specialise in community work are undoubtedly going to be able to offer people who have a serious mental disorder or handicap a service highly sensitive to their particular needs.

Those needs are often complex and they require a flexible approach. So it is sensible for community psychiatric nurses to continue to work in multi-disciplinary specialist teams. The same applies to community mental handicap nurses. At a time when services are already undergoing radical change as a result of the shift from institutional to community care, we do not feel it is right to suggest organisational or managerial changes which could sever those links.

A welcome trend has been the attachment of community psychiatric nurses and community mental handicap nurses to primary health care teams or to health visiting and district nursing services. The opportunity for community psychiatric nurses and community mental handicap nurses to share community premises can strengthen the relationship between specialist services and primary health care services. To ensure they continue to contribute to primary care, the neighbourhood nursing manager and managers of community psychiatric and community mental handicap nurses should agree the respective roles the specialists and other community nurses will play in meeting the needs of people with mental handicap or mental health problems.

We learned that an obstacle to the development of
community psychiatric nursing and community mental
handicap nursing is the threat to the mental health
officer status of nurses when they become community-
based. This is a matter for the Whitley Council, but we
hope it can ensure that psychiatric and mental handicap
nurses with mental health officer status when based in
hospital are not disadvantaged when they take up
community work.

Other specialist nurses

The remaining group consists mainly of registered
general nurses who, from a base in the community or from
a hospital, have developed a special interest, often
after additional training. They include stoma care
nurses, diabetic nurse specialists, continence advisers,
nurses for terminally ill people, and health visitors
for elderly people. These nurses are normally but not
always managed as part of community nursing services.
It is when they are based in hospital and are managed as
part of the hospital service that problems most often
occur in co-ordinating their work with that of community
nurses.

In the light of what we have described,

WE RECOMMEND that

> **Community midwives, community psychiatric nurses
> and community mental handicap nurses should
> ensure, through their respective managers and the
> neighbourhood nursing manager, that their
> specialist contributions are fully co-ordinated
> with the work of the neighbourhood nursing
> service.**

As neighbourhood nursing services become established and
existing professional roles become blurred, we would
expect relationships to change. We would like to see in
five years' time a fundamental review of the needs of
the clients of these specialists and of how the services
provided for them could be further improved.

WE RECOMMEND also that

> **All other specialist nurses who work outside**

hospital should be based in the community and
managed as part of the neighbourhood nursing
service. Each specialist nurse should be
assigned to one or more neighbourhood services
and have the commitment of her time to each
service specified.

In all cases they should aim to co-ordinate their work
with neighbourhood nurses and other care agencies, such
as Macmillan nurses, so that when more than one care
giver is involved with an individual or family a key
worker can be identified. If a family already has
regular contact with a community nurse, the specialist
nurse should aim to work through her. She should help
her at the same time to develop her skills: it is a
waste of valuable resources if specialised nurses work
exclusively to particular patients in the community
rather than transfer at least some of their skills to
nurses already working in the community.

The neighbourhood nursing service should be kept
informed about the work and role of specialist nurses
and of their specialist teams, and should always have
access to them so that everyone understands their
respective roles, the level of demand for services and
the kind of support clients need.

7:NEW ROLES

Specialist nurses should, by example and by sharing their knowledge with other staff, encourage individual health visitors, district nurses and school nurses to develop special interests of their own in response to consumer needs.

We could envisage, for example, a health visitor developing advanced skills in the recognition and handling of child abuse, another specialising in child development, a district nurse developing expertise in the care of dying people and another in counselling on family or marital problems. Nurses could develop such interests without abandoning their more general workloads, working on a sessional basis in clinics or in the home or as part-time members of short-life task forces set up to tackle particular problems, such as identifying and helping homeless and rootless people. They could also consider, with their managers, the possibility of becoming nurse practitioners.

The nurse practitioner

The concept of the nurse practitioner in primary health care was commended to us by several of the organisations which gave evidence.

In this country, nurse practitioners are rare. We believe that community nurses who have, or acquire, the necessary skills in health promotion and the diagnosis and treatment of disease among people of all ages should have the opportunity to practise those skills in the setting of a clinic in the neighbourhood.

We are not proposing they should become mini-doctors. We are suggesting that patients who visit their general practitioners with conditions which are self-limiting, or want to discuss another aspect of their health care, should have a choice of whom to see. Research has shown that nurses can be as effective as doctors - and as acceptable to patients - in securing compliance with therapy for chronic disease, making initial assessments of patients, diagnosing and treating certain minor acute illnesses and behavioural disorders, and rehabilitating elderly people after surgery.

We considered whether in each primary health care team of requisite size one community nurse should be encouraged to take on the role of a "nurse practitioner". We also considered whether to recommend that this role should automatically be made a career grade for experienced nurses wanting to continue in clinical practice. However, we saw certain disadvantages:

> More than one nurse in a team might be suitably qualified and experienced to act as a nurse practitioner.

> We would prefer all community nurses to be able to receive and deal with referrals direct from the public; the creation of a nurse practitioner grade might confuse this principle.

> The career grade principle should apply to other roles as and when warranted.

The view we took, therefore, was that where a primary health care team agrees it is appropriate to provide the kind of service we have described, it should be on the basis of a set number of clinic sessions each week to be taken by whichever nurse, or nurses, are qualified to perform the role.

WE RECOMMEND that

> **The principle should be adopted of introducing the nurse practitioner into primary health care.**

Subject to the agreement of local general practitioners, the nurse practitioner should be assigned for an agreed minimum of hours each week to either a single general practitioner or group of general practitioners. She should be managed by the neighbourhood nursing manager and be responsible to the general practitioner(s) for carrying out agreed medical protocols.

Her key tasks would be to interview patients and diagnose and treat specific diseases in accordance with the agreed medical protocols; refer to the general practitioner patients who have medical problems which lie outside the written protocols; be available for all patients who wish to consult the nurse practitioner; give counselling and nursing advice to patients consulting her direct or referred to her by a general practitioner; conduct screening programmes among specific age- or client-groups; maintain patient-care programmes, particularly to the chronic sick; refer patients for further nursing care to the neighbourhood nursing service.

Special responsibilities for managers

Neighbourhood nursing managers and senior nurse managers should also be able to develop special interests and take on specific additional functions. These might include: the co-ordination and development of the health authority's policy and practice regarding children at risk of abuse or neglect; liaison with local authority social service and education departments; liaison with hospitals on service planning; inspection of nursing homes licensed by the health authority; and giving professional advice to local polytechnics or colleges of higher education on nurse education and research matters.

Power to prescribe

We found district nurses waste time in requesting prescriptions from general practitioners for such things as dressings, ointments and medical sprays - those for leg ulcers, for example.

In addition, many nurses have become very skilled in managing pain relief programmes for terminally ill patients. We believe therefore that community nurses who work with terminally ill patients should be permitted to use their professional judgement on matters such as the timing and dosage of drugs prescribed for pain relief.

WE RECOMMEND that

> **The DHSS should agree a limited list of items and simple agents which may be prescribed by nurses as part of a nursing care programme, and issue guidelines to enable nurses to control drug dosage in well-defined circumstances.**

Detailed medical protocols should be drawn up with general practitioners which encourage community nurses within strictly agreed limits to vary the timing and

dosage and use of alternative pain relief agents for
patients who have been diagnosed by general
practitioners as terminally ill and in pain. This may
require nurses carrying their own small supply of drugs,
as midwives do now.

8: IMPROVING PRIMARY CARE TEAMWORK

Neighbourhood nursing services should not be seen as substitutes for primary health care teams. They should be seen as a comprehensive reinforcement where primary health care teams already exist. Where such teams do not exist, however, the neighbourhood nursing service would be a cogent and clearly recognisable agency for the provision of health care in association with general practitioners. To reinforce and promote good teamwork we believe that a formal agreement between general practitioners and neighbourhood nursing services would be an important key to the effective delivery of primary care services.

WE RECOMMEND therefore that

> To establish and be recognised as a primary health care team, each general medical practice and the community nurses associated with it should come to an understanding of the team's objectives and individuals' roles within it.

> That understanding should be incorporated into a written agreement signed jointly by the practice partners and by the manager of the neighbourhood nursing service on behalf of the relevant health authority.

> The agreement should name the doctors and community nurses who together form the primary care team and should guarantee the right of the team members to be consulted on any changes proposed in its composition.

> The making of such an agreement should be a qualifying condition for any incentive payments which may be introduced to improve quality in general practice (as suggested in the recent policy statement of the Royal College of General Practitioners).

We think there would be value in having a written agreement which could be referred to readily. We believe there would be positive advantages for doctors, because they would be assured of support from a team of nurses who would be known to them.

Changes in the membership of the team would not be possible without prior consultation with the doctors by the neighbourhood nursing manager. They would be involved in decisions about the development and extension of the nurses' role and be able to exert influence on policies for the provision of nursing services to the communities in which they work. Teams founded on such an agreement would prove to be attractive centres around which paramedical and other specialist services would be organised.

They would also be centres to which universities and colleges of higher education would want to send students for practical experience, and would become teaching practices in the real sense of the term for both community nurses and doctors.

Doctors who preferred not to negotiate such an agreement would receive only those nursing services which the neighbourhood nursing managers themselves decide to provide. In the absence of a joint agreement, we would expect the nursing manager to give the general practitioners concerned a written statement of what those services would be. No guarantee could be given in such circumstances that the practice would always have the same group of nurses to deal with their referrals.

We suggest in the Programme for Action the points we would expect such agreements to cover. Each agreement would need to make clear the basis on which nurses would be available (for example, if not whole-time, the number of hours or number of clinic sessions a week they would work); their scope to deal directly with self-referrals from the public for nursing care and health advice; and the medical and nursing protocol for deciding the appropriate course of action to take on receiving referrals (including the rights of nurses to refer cases on to other nurses).

Disseminating good practice

We believe agreements on the lines we have described would be an important stimulus to improvement and lead to a better service for the consumer. Improvements, where they happen, tend not, however, to be broadcast very widely, if at all.

It became more and more clear to us, as we visited

Districts and studied evidence, that little or no
systematic attempt is made to share knowledge and
experience of good practice in primary care. We saw
unco-ordinated effort by hard-pressed health workers who
were developing imaginative and effective schemes,
believing them to be unique, only to find similar
schemes mirrored in other Districts nearby.

We were asked on many occasions to list examples of good
practice which we encountered. Among the shining
examples we came across were:

> District nurses running a hospital-at-home
> scheme; health visitors fostering self-reliance
> in parents in disadvantaged families through
> structured visiting; psychiatric nurse therapists
> working within the primary health care team; a
> community unit joining forces with a local
> authority social service department to run a
> dusk, night and dawn service to support carers
> and those dependent on them; an off-peak health
> visiting service where the health visitors, in
> addition to responding to families' phone
> enquiries, run evening groups and health sessions
> and do home visits; a community mental handicap
> team which had interviewed the parents of all the
> handicapped children in its area to identify
> present needs; a primary health care team with
> excellent aims and objectives and evaluation of
> its health care delivery.

Schemes like these should be more widely known. The
effective dissemination of good practice can lead to
higher standards of service. We gave some thought to
the possibility of suggesting the creation of a national
accreditation body which might monitor standards and
spread good practice. We decided, however, that this
would probably be too bureaucratic and costly.

Instead, WE RECOMMEND that

> **The Government should invite the Health Advisory
> Service, with its established reputation,
> credibility and acceptance by the professions, to
> take on responsibility for identifying and
> promoting good practice in primary health care.**

The HAS already takes an interest in some aspects of

primary care, but we appreciate that its terms of reference would have to be extended beyond the present remit for elderly people and mentally ill people. We have no doubt that with adequate resources the HAS would be willing and well able to widen its scope to cover all aspects of primary health care.

9:PRACTICE NURSES

We were asked to consider the position and contribution
of nurses directly employed by general practitioners.
They are mostly known as practice nurses. We heard from
many individual practice nurses and general
practitioners about why doctors employ their own nurses.
It is mainly because they feel unable to obtain from the
local health authority the services of a nurse to be
employed on duties they want carried out.

It is our view that, as neighbourhood nursing services
develop, as the basis for primary care teamwork is made
clear through written agreements with general
practitioners, and as nurses take on new roles such as
that of the nurse practitioner, general practitioners
should have less and less reason or wish to employ their
own nursing staff.

Several authorities, through their nurse management
organisation, have put restrictions on the duties which
can be carried out by district nurses and health
visitors. This may be because the managers judge that
there are not enough nurses to undertake all the work
required or because work undertaken in general
practitioners' surgeries is seen as secondary to the
main work of district nursing and health visiting staff.
Managers and nurses may also object to undertaking work
in general practitioners' premises, such as vaccination
and immunisation, for which the doctors are entitled to
- and claim - items-of-service payments for the
practice.

The figures for England available from the DHSS show
that over the past ten years the number of practice
nurses employed by general practitioners has grown
rapidly. In 1974 there were more than 1,000 practice
nurses. In 1984 there were nearly 4,000, mostly working
part-time for an average of about 18 hours a week. The
increase has become steeper in the last five years with
the number of nurses doubling in that period.

Under the general practitioners' ancillary staff scheme,
doctors can be reimbursed for 70 per cent of the
salaries of some of the staff they employ. These staff
can include nurses. With tax concessions, the weekly
cost to a general practitioner employing a nurse for ten

hours is less than £8. It is not altogether surprising, therefore, that the number of nurses employed by general practitioners has increased so sharply. A recent article in the British Medical Journal demonstrated how, through judicious use of the items-of-service payments scheme - for example, having the nurse carry out a few innoculations - a general practitioners' practice is able easily to cover the nurse's salary costs.

We recognise the good work many practice nurses are doing, but we believe that in financial terms the arrangements give very uncertain value for money - to the consumer especially - if they are allowed to continue in the present uncontrolled way. If all doctors took up their entitlement, the number of practice nurses would soar by 20,000. This would cost the NHS more than £100 million a year and start to drain the pool of nursing staff available for duties which health authorities consider as priorities.

We believe that through the setting-up of neighbourhood nursing services, general practitioners would be able to get from health authorities the nurses they require to carry out treatments and other nursing work in their premises. Continued reliance on large numbers of directly employed nurses, on the other hand, could damage the cohesion of the neighbourhood nursing services.

WE RECOMMEND therefore that

> **Subsidies to general practitioners enabling them to employ staff to perform nursing duties should be phased out.**

We recognise there would be an additional cost to health authorities if they are to be expected to provide the nurses required to work in general practitioners' surgeries. It is not unreasonable to expect, however, that some of the family practitioner service funds which go towards subsidising general practitioners could be transferred to the DHSS Community Health Account. We estimate that in England more than £10 million is paid each year by the Government to general practitioners to employ their own nurses. Whatever the immediate cost implications of ending the subsidy, we believe this is a necessary step if this potentially excessive demand on family practitioner service finances is to be controlled.

We have great sympathy with the view expressed to us by the Royal College of Nursing that, as a matter of professional principle, nurses should not be subject to control and direction by doctors over their professional work.

The College suggested that doctors generally do not arrange appropriate training for nursing staff; and the staff lack the professional nursing support which is often required. The result is that consumers get a fragmented and less than adequate clinical nursing service. "Consumers, nurses and general practitioners deserve something better", said the College.

If, despite this, general practitioners still wish to employ their own nurses, and nurses wish to work for them, nothing we propose stops this happening. General practitioners, as independent contractors, are businessmen. If for them it makes business sense to employ a nurse, even without a subsidy, that, we recognise, remains their prerogative.

10:IMPLICATIONS FOR TRAINING

There are short- and long-term implications for training in our proposals. In the short-term, time and resources would need to be invested in preparing people for the establishment of neighbourhood nursing services, helping managers and nurses to work effectively as teams, helping them to identify needs in the communities they serve, tap into and build up the informal networks of support which already exist, use management information to question the way they work now, and develop new roles and working relationships. We consider the question of "resources for change" in Section 12.

Our proposals for bringing district nurses, health visitors, school nurses and other nurses working in the community together into neighbourhood nursing services would we believe, have a major impact on the way nurses are trained in these fields.

The training and education of health visitors, district nurses and school nurses have improved in recent years. But, despite the potential this gives them for developing their roles and widening the services they can give consumers, we found that in practice they are still hemmed inside their own disciplines. We want to see them use their skills to the full, developing them according to their particular interests and the demands for help which can be anticipated or occur in their particular neighbourhood.

The neighbourhood nursing service offers the means for change. As a further means to promote that change,

WE RECOMMEND that

> **Within two years the United Kingdom Central Council for Nursing, Midwifery and Health Visiting and the English National Board should introduce a common training course for all first-level nurses wishing to work outside hospital in what are now the fields of health visiting, district nursing and school nursing.**

Successful completion of the course should lead to the qualification of a Diploma in Community Nursing and Health Care.

We would see such a course following the broad basis of the present health visiting course, developed to take account of the wider requirements of all nurses wishing to work in the community.

The diploma course would be undertaken in universities and colleges of higher education in exactly the same way as existing health visitors' courses are held. It should last one academic year, after which the nurse would work for a further year under supervision.

The supervision period would consist of a planned programme of experience over the whole range of community health care. Successful completion of this supervised practice period, together with completion of a specialist module, would lead to the issuing of an ENB certificate suitably endorsed with the specialist module. This in turn should lead, we suggest, to registration on the health visitor part of the Professional Register.

Specialist modules would cover one of several options such as maternal and child health, home nursing, health care of adolescents and young children, mental health care, health education, nurse practitioner work, or occupational health.

Part-time and evening sessions, as well as full-time day courses, should be made available so that a maximum number of staff may be involved. Distance-learning packages could also be provided. In this way, community nurses could take further specialist modules.

For the full impact of the new training to take effect, we think it essential that conversion courses should be provided to enable existing qualified community nurses to broaden their skills in the same way as new entrants. There would need to be safeguards to protect the position of existing nurses who would qualify for such training but might not be allowed by a health authority to take the course because funds or replacement staff were not available. In district nursing, this was overcome by the DHSS in 1981 requiring health authorities to offer the appropriate nine-month course to those involved within five years. We believe that five years would be a reasonable timescale.

We would encourage statutory bodies to set up courses leading to a higher diploma in nursing and health care and to a Masters' Degree. This would encourage a greater study of community health and equip some nurses to plan services in more depth than has been possible before.

We must emphasise that we are not proposing the introduction of a generic nurse, but we do see common training as the one way to break down the rigid roles these nurses have at present. We are seeking to preserve the type of skills possessed by the health visitor and to create more scope for her to practise them. We are also seeking to heighten and widen opportunities for district nurses and school nurses. At last, they would be able, individually and as team members, to take a far more flexible approach to their clients and patients and to treat them not as so many separate parts but as whole people - in whole neighbourhoods.

We make no firm recommendation about the title by which nurses who complete the proposed common training should be known. We would favour something straightforward, such as "community health nurse", but we recognise that this would be for the professional and training bodies to decide.

Psychiatric and mental handicap nursing

We considered whether to recommend that the common training course should be even broader based to cater for **all** first-level nurses wishing to work in the community - that is, for nurses wishing to work with people who have mental health problems or a mental handicap as well as for those wishing to work in the fields already mentioned. We decided against this, mainly because we felt the time is not right.

We recognise that basic training courses for psychiatric and mental handicap nurses have developed considerably in recent years and that with the introduction of the syllabuses agreed in 1982 we can expect still further developments, with a much greater emphasis on community care than before.

Our first concern has been to ensure that suitably trained community nurses are provided to form the core

of the neighbourhood nursing service. We have said that
for the time being community psychiatric and mental
handicap nurses should not be core members, but that
they should nevertheless work closely with the
neighbourhood nursing service with a view eventually to
becoming integrated. As these services become
established we would expect working relationships to
become stronger.

We have therefore suggested (Section 6) that in five
years' time there should be a fundamental review of how
nursing services provided outside hospital to meet the
needs of people with mental health problems or a mental
handicap could be further improved. That is the time
for the statutory training bodies to consider whether
one common training course for all nurses wishing to
work in the community is appropriate.

We believe, however, that steps could be taken by the
training bodies in the meantime to facilitate the close
working relationships we wish to see. It should be
possible to identify elements in community psychiatric
and community mental handicap training courses which
could also form part of the new common training course
we recommend. For these elements we would urge the
training bodies to provide opportunities for shared
learning.

We believe that specific education and training courses
are required for psychiatric and mental handicap nurses
working in the community and that satisfactory
completion of such courses ought to be a prerequisite to
practise. We are concerned, therefore, with the low
level of uptake of the relevant courses currently
provided by the ENB. The position needs to be kept
under close review by the ENB and health authorities in
the light of our recommendations.

Enrolled nurses

Neighbourhood nursing managers would need to explore
carefully the balance of skill levels required in their
staff, and the extent to which highly trained nurses
would be necessary for the effective delivery of care.
Although our emphasis in this section has been on the
training required by first-level nurses we still see a
need for enrolled nurses in the community. We would
therefore strongly urge the statutory training bodies

to ensure that suitable educational and training courses
are continued and developed to prepare enrolled nurses
to undertake work in the community as part of
neighbourhood nursing services, under the direction of
fully qualified community nurses.

11:FUTURE MANAGEMENT OF COMMUNITY NURSING SERVICES

In considering people's needs, and how organisationally they can best be met, we examined whether district health authorities should continue to have responsibility for providing nursing services in the community. The desire for change and improvement was strong, particularly among the nursing professions' representative bodies, and we were offered a number of radical proposals. One of the most radical was to put all primary health care under the control of one authority. For example, it was suggested to us that family practitioner committees could be turned into primary health care authorities with strong nursing representation in determining policies, allocation of resources and planning of services.

We could not ignore, however, the voices of many nurses and their managers who, already unnerved by Griffiths-inspired changes in NHS management, told us that any further fundamental changes in organisation were needed (as one put it bluntly) "like a hole in the head".

We had sympathy with this view. The NHS reorganisation of 1974 brought community and hospital nursing services together. We were not convinced that to separate them again would be in the best interests of consumers, particularly bearing in mind the increasing emphasis on earlier discharge of acute hospital patients into the community, the development of day surgery and the potential for hospital-at-home schemes.

The Department of Health's Standing Nursing and Midwifery Advisory Committee, which "believes strongly" that community nurses should still be employed by district health authorities, added that the continued integration of nursing services must include satisfactory planning, resource allocation and training opportunities. We agree wholeheartedly with that, and believe district health authorities are best placed to provide them.

Another equally radical proposal we considered was to merge family practitioner committees and health authorities, and to add all general practitioners and other primary health care workers to the payroll of the merged authorities - either directly by making primary care a salaried service or indirectly by contracting out primary care to doctors and nurses working as a business partnership.

In our informal discussions with health care professionals, the idea that general practitioners might one day become salaried was not completely discounted, and we met some individual general practitioners who, like us, see advantages in such arrangements: primary health care would be brought firmly and uncompromisingly into the strategic planning framework of a single health authority, there would be clearer lines of accountability by all primary health care workers and there would be integrated control of financial and manpower resources. This would make sense for everyone, not least the consumer.

For the immediate future we reluctantly rejected the idea. This was partly because of the recent upheavals in the organisation and management of family practitioner committees and district health authorities, which must be given a chance to settle down, and partly because we believe such a measure would be summarily rejected by family practitioners at this time. We hope, nevertheless, that the idea is not entirely lost sight of in the future.

We also considered suggestions that community nurses, as well as practice nurses, should be employed by general practitioners. This could conceivably lead to better teamwork, but the weight of evidence we received was against such an arrangement for various reasons, some of which we have referred to in Section 9. A frequently heard comment of nurses was that general practitioners' work is concerned largely with the diagnosis and treatment of illness and that this would sooner or later pervade the working attitudes and behaviour of their nursing staff to the detriment of preventive care and health promotion.

There is also the danger, we were told, that nurses might be subordinated to the roles of "handmaidens" to the doctors. We do not believe that in enlightened and progressive practices this would happen, but we do believe that, even in well-run, highly motivated practices, the employment of the community nurses by general practitioners would make it impossible to ensure a round-the-clock nursing service which a health authority, with more flexible use of greater resources, is capable of providing and which we think is essential.

We finally considered the idea of offering community nursing services back to local authorities. This was virtually a non-starter. None of the local authority organisations we heard from supported the idea, except on the grounds of coterminosity of health and social services. We were given the clear impression that most local authorities had enough on their plates without adding health services to them again.

We decided community nursing services should stay where they are - with district health authorities - and we have concentrated on how they can most efficiently and effectively be provided in conjunction with general practitioner services.

WE RECOMMEND therefore that

> **The provision of nursing services in the community should remain the responsibility of district health authorities. We would urge, however, that in due course the Government should give consideration to amalgamating family practitioner committees and district health authorities and so bring all primary health care services under the control of one body.**

Nursing management structure

Each neighbourhood nursing service and its manager should be part of a clearly identified and practical management structure in each health authority. A neighbourhood nursing service covering a population in the middle of the range of 10,000 and 25,000 would typically consist of about ten qualified community nurses. With three or four other qualified staff or auxiliaries, it is a viable management unit.

It is not unusual, under existing management arrangements, for a community nursing manager to have more than 30 staff reporting directly to her. Even without allowing for the scattered base of working this is an exceptional span of control: it is like having all hospital ward nurses reporting directly to a nursing officer without a ward sister in between.

For the organisation we propose to work effectively, the neighbourhood nursing manager should ideally be responsible for no more than 15 staff and in turn to have a senior nursing manager whom she can approach readily for professional advice and support. The senior nursing manager should normally have no more than ten neighbourhood nursing managers reporting to her. Where a District consists of more than ten neighbourhoods, it would probably be desirable to group them into two (or more) broad sectors to ensure that proper control and direction could be exercised. Heads of such sectors should be graded and paid at a level appropriate to their managerial responsibilities.

Given the enormous range in size, style and composition of the new general management units, and the similar variations which are bound to occur in each neighbourhood nursing service, it would be wrong for us to be prescriptive about the detailed managerial structures, except to say there should be:

> clear management lines,

> limited spans of control,

> integration with wider unit management arrangements.

This should enable managers to be fully responsible for the deployment and control of resources identified at each level. Once sufficient information on activities and finances can be provided management budgets should be held by the neighbourhood nursing managers.

We offer, purely as an example, the structure which might apply in an average-sized District. This would have 15 neighbourhoods. Each neighbourhood nursing service would consist of eight to 12 qualified community nurses and three to four other staff. The total staffing might be:

	Current	Proposed
Director/Assistant director	1	2
Nurse manager	8	15
District nurses, health visitors, school nurses	135	130
Other fieldwork staff	56	56
	200	203

Half the 15 neighbourhood nursing managers would probably have medium to small neighbourhoods and would be able to undertake direct clinical work, in which case the total qualified fieldwork staff would remain about the same.

12:<u>RESOURCES FOR CHANGE</u>

Our proposals not only involve changes of emphasis in the delivery of care and style of management; they may also mean the planned and deliberate diversion of resources. How this might be achieved would largely be a matter for local decision; we can do no more than indicate the areas in which new costs would be incurred, and how resources might be released to cover them.

The information on manpower and its costs available to us from the DHSS was unclear. As we said earlier, there has been some growth in the numbers of community nursing staff and a change in the skill mix. The precise nature and underlying cause for these changes cannot, however, be determined from the very limited data available. Nor can any reliable projection be made.

We have resisted pressure from several quarters to suggest norms of provision. Even if better information were available centrally we do not believe national norms should be promulgated. Our whole approach is concerned with identifying and responding to neighbourhood needs, and therefore staff levels should be decided locally in the light of local requirements and priorities.

From the limited evidence and from the recent trends in staffing levels, it was impossible to assess with accuracy how far the supply of staff satisfies demand. Regional plans for community services suggest that the demand nationally is likely to grow at a lower rate overall in the future than in recent years.

Only in a few areas of the country does recruitment of staff appear difficult. Recruitment for health visiting does not generally appear to be a major problem; one authority had 200 applicants for seven health visitor training places. The recruitment of district nurses is more difficult. One District reported ten vacancies in an establishment of 36, a result of which was that it was unable to provide a full 24-hour nursing service it was planning. In the present economic climate, many vacant posts are being frozen or cut from establishments. Five authorities alone in London reported this. The UKCC reported that the secondment pattern of health authorities at present appears to be based on maintaining establishments and not on the development of a community nursing service to meet local health needs.

Concern was expressed to us about the shortage of places for district nurse training since mandatory training has been introduced. One health authority reported that registered general nurses were waiting two to three years to be given college places. In the case of health visitors, the problem is that some courses are being curtailed because of the restriction on health visitor sponsorship. We hope that both matters will be looked at by the ENB and the health authorities.

The questions of retention of staff and high turnover rates were highlighted in the inner cities - for example, in London where the annual turnover rates for district nurses was between 13.5 per cent and 40 per cent and for health visitors between 14.7 per cent and 28 per cent. Measures taken to tackle this problem could include the development of a career grade for community nurses, more flexibility over work sharing and the employment of part-time staff, the provision of better working conditions, and the availability of peer group support from other professionals.

The prospects for such changes would be enhanced through the improved management structure we propose and by the introduction of new personal review and appraisal systems.

However the work of district nurses, health visitors and other nurses working in the community is carried out in the future, and especially in the longer term, it is essential to ensure the right numbers of skilled staff are available.

In view of the confusing picture which exists,

WE RECOMMEND that

A short but thorough manpower planning exercise on a practical (as distinct from purely academic) basis should be undertaken to ensure that the training and supply of community nurses is, and remains at, the appropriate level. The study should be supported by the NHS Management Board

**as an essential task in reviewing the adequacy
and consistency of Regional plans.**

As part of the exercise it will be essential to
estimate recruitment and leaving rates in order to
understand the dynamics of the staffing position as well
as the current manpower picture.

Although the detailed picture is unclear at the moment,
we believe the changes we propose in the organisation of
community nursing services can and should be made.
There is now a mood and momentum for change which must
be built upon. However, to ensure success we believe
strongly that resources should be invested in the
process of change. They are needed in three ways.

Training needs

Firstly, deliberate efforts must be made to set up and
finance appropriate training courses. Health
authorities have a responsibility to see that their
employees - nurses and auxiliaries - are trained to do
the work they are paid for. We noted with concern wide
contrasts in the financing of in-service training. In
some authorities it is generous, in others extremely
poor. The use of local resources is to be encouraged,
but community nurses should be able, and indeed
encouraged, to attend national courses. It should also
be possible to "buy in" expert help. Where training is
centrally planned and budgeted for, the senior nurse
manager should ensure that the training needs of the
community nurses are well represented.

Extra resources would also be required to finance the
new shared training we propose for health visitors,
district nurses and school nurses, and any conversion or
updating courses which might be established. We have
not attempted to cost them in detail; the costs would
depend on the action taken as a result of our proposals
and on up-to-date information on staff recruitment,
retention and turnover. We urge the DHSS to do this
with the UKCC, ENB and health authorities in the same
way it has attempted to identify the cost implications
of the changes recently proposed by the ENB in basic
nurse training.

Management changes

Secondly, extra resources would probably be needed for the strengthening we propose of the management of community nursing services. In our view, this is a vital investment.

Using the illustration on page 51, we estimate that the total additional salary cost to an average health authority of the arrangements could be about £35,000 a year - or less than two per cent of current expenditure. We believe the benefits of the improved control and direction of resources which the new arrangements would bring would far outweigh the cost.

Pay and rewards

The third issue concerns the pay and rewards available for nurses. The Royal College of General Practitioners said in its evidence: "Financial and professional rewards should ensure that the best nurses and health visitors continue in clinical practice if they so choose; these nurses should give new leadership within practice teams and should set the pace for high standards in nursing practice and in teaching by their personal example." This is in line with comments made by, among others, the Royal College of Nursing and the Health Visitors' Association, and we very much endorse this view.

Senior nurse salary scales offer a framework which in some parts of the country is used imaginatively to enable highly skilled community nurses to follow a clinical career path instead of having to go into main-line management simply because that is where the financial rewards or status are. We hope health authorities will ensure every opportunity and incentive is offered to nurses to develop their careers in client care services and to be properly remunerated for it. The senior nursing grades used need not be included in management cost assessments and therefore should not require monitoring by regional health authorities.

We considered whether, in order to ensure that funds are made available for this purpose, a central reserve should be created by the Government. We had in mind the so-called "Acheson" money set aside by the DHSS in 1983 for a four-year period to improve primary care in the inner cities. We believe, however, most health authorities would be against further top-slicing of the total amount of revenue advances available to the NHS to do this. In the absence of such a fund we would urge the NHS Management Board and regional health authorities to encourage district health authorities to make imaginative use of their community health service budgets to provide nurses with appropriate incentives.

Finding the resources

We have noted from their strategic plans that, as a result of deliberate efforts by community nursing services to support patients at home, several regional health authorities anticipate overall reductions in lengths of in-patient hospital stay and in the total numbers of acute beds over the next decade. We applaud the philosophy of care this reflects, but if the changes planned are to be carried through in practice, it is crucial that the savings are transferred to the community sector and not absorbed into developing new, more highly specialised forms of hospital care. The District Nursing Association called for "stronger advocacy for the unglamorous side of community nursing (which) all too often, in competition with the more costly hospital care, takes a back seat."

In some cases, no change in the use of beds will be possible unless some form of bridging finance is made available to help build up the community nursing services first. We hope the Management Board will pay particular attention to this issue as part of its task of monitoring the implementation by health authorities of their declared policies.

We believe considerable scope and potential exist for virement between hospital and community budgets. As an example, we found in one District that the service provided by paediatric home nurses had a definite impact on the use made of hospital beds for children. By helping parents to nurse chronically ill children at home, the service had prevented unnecessary admissions to hospital and had helped to reduce by half the frequency and average lengths of stay of those who were admitted. But we found no evidence that there had been a shift of resources as a result. We also saw schemes run by community nurses to provide respite care for frail elderly people, thus, again, preventing unnecessary admission to hospital.

The effects of virement between hospital and community budgets on the balance of care can be very marked for community nursing. Between 1983 and 1984, for example, the average length of stay in acute hospitals decreased by 0.3 days. At existing cost rates and throughput this is equivalent to a "saving" of £130 million.

Transferring this sum entirely to the community nursing services, which must bear extra workload for earlier discharge of patients, would enable an extra 75 qualified community nurses to be employed in each District - an increase of about one third. Put another way, for the cost of providing a service to patients in one bed in an acute hospital in a year - about £25,000 - approximately two-and-a-half community nurses could be employed and provide a daily visit to 15 patients or a weekly visit to 75 patients during every week of the year. Hence, as the balance of hospital work changes, it presents both the need and the opportunity to make striking improvements to community nursing levels.

We would expect, too, savings to be found as a result of neighbourhood nursing services having better management information and looking critically at their current practices. For example, a health visitor visits a pre-school child just under four times a year. If these visits were generally more selective and reduced by, say, 25 per cent, the equivalent of about 1,500 health visitors would be available for work with other client groups: it would, for example, allow the amount of time spent with elderly people to be increased to two-and-a-half times its present level.

More resources could also be freed by improved organisation, support and management. A prime target must be travelling time and costs. A 1980 survey of nurses' work indicated that 16 per cent of health visitors' time and 24 per cent of district nurses' time was spent on travel. The neighbourhood-based organisation we have proposed should reduce this. It could also be reduced through better management control and direction, by community nurses making advance appointments with their clients, and by encouraging people to visit health centres rather than receive domiciliary visits.

Reducing travel time for all nursing staff by ten per cent would free up resources equivalent to two per cent of current staff - incidentally, the same as the total salary increase envisaged on page 55 for the management and staffing structure illustrated earlier.

Many community nurses remarked to us on the large amount of time spent on clerical and administrative tasks, and the 1980 survey supported their concern by showing that nearly 15 per cent of district nurses' time and 25 per cent of health visitors' time is spent in this way. In an average District this costs more than £250,000 a year for qualified staff alone. There is therefore scope through the introduction of improved procedures, including computerisation, and extra clerical assistance to make cost-effective changes. If the employment of one clerk could reduce the amount of clerical time spent by qualified staff by 20 per cent, net savings could be achieved or additional professional service given.

In striving to improve the quality and quantity of service given by community nurses there is enormous scope for achievement even without additional resources. We believe the more concentrated, directed and responsive management style we propose could help to bring this about.

13:THE CONSUMER'S CONTRIBUTION

Our report has been about the organisation, management and development of community nursing services and primary health care. We have drawn a broad picture of people's health care needs, but it would be in the neighbourhoods themselves that the details of needs would be highlighted and wherever possible responded to. This is not a job only for the professionals; it is something in which the consumers themselves should play a part.

If health authorities and health professionals are to take the interests of the consumer seriously, there needs to be a forum where local people can contribute their views on health needs and health care planning. We recognise the important role community health councils already take in this activity, but, like district health authorities, they can be remote from the neighbourhoods we envisage.

We learned of many successful collaborative ventures involving the public, statutory and voluntary bodies, and community nurses. Many neighbourhoods, especially those in areas with traditions of self-help, are able to harness support, energy and influence to achieve results for schemes which will benefit the health of the community.

The energy and impetus come from different sources, and much of their success stems from the enthusiasm and commitment of individuals. But enthusiasm and commitment are not always enough. Nor are they always directed at the right targets. We would like to see positive encouragement from health authorities for the creation of community groups which would stimulate and channel action in response to local needs which have so far gone unrecognised or unmet.

The mechanism for this would vary from place to place but, as an example,

WE RECOMMEND that

> **Health care associations should be formed, each covering one or more neighbourhoods.**

The associations, constituted as local people think best, could be established by local groups, the community health council, the health care professionals or the health authority - or any combination of them.

Membership would vary according to the character and perceived needs of the locality, but it would be essential for CHCs, with their wealth of experience in dealing with health authorities and in consumer advocacy, to be represented. The associations should certainly include the neighbourhood nursing manager and ideally a general practitioner. Representatives from education, social services, housing and voluntary organisations should be co-opted as and when appropriate.

A health care association should be compact and not become a mini-bureaucracy. Small groups already exist which are getting things done because they are small and dynamic. They also have the capacity to generate resources of money and people simply because they are seen to be dealing with perceived neighbourhood needs.

Health care associations would meet regularly to identify problems and needs and consider how best action might be taken by statutory and voluntary agencies to deal with them.

With the health care professionals, they should help to publicise neighbourhood primary care and nursing services and guide people on how and where to obtain advice and help.

People living in the neighbourhood should be informed how they can influence decisions on the way services are provided and how they can complain if they are dissatisfied. The way this information is presented can influence the public's perception of the services and their take-up of them, and therefore we would expect health care associations, and the health authorities generally, to seek expert publicity and marketing advice.

The public's ideas and opinions on the development of local services might be obtained through public seminars, smaller semi-structured discussions with users of particular services, regular patient participation groups associated with a doctor's practice, and local voluntary organisations which take on the role of advocate for particular groups of consumers - for example, people whose first language is not English.

More participation in "good health" programmes - for example, to improve diet, reduce smoking, encourage physical exercise and foster mental health - is needed if the quality of individual lifestyles is to be enhanced and if the NHS is to cope with the rising costs and expectations of a population ill-prepared for maturity and old age.

"Participation" was a word we heard frequently during our discussions. So, too, was the word "partnership".

The need for partnership was emphasised particularly strongly by the consumers themselves as represented by the Association of Community Health Councils in England and Wales. They told us: "It is important to generate an ethos among nurses and other professionals which would lead them to regard patients or clients, families and friends, as partners in the caring exercise. Granted that many appear to welcome dependency and traditional nursing attitudes encourage it, involvement, personal responsibility and participation would seem to be more appropriate."

We echo that.

SUMMARY OF RECOMMENDATIONS

1   Each district health authority should identify within
    its boundaries neighbourhoods for the purposes of
    planning, organising and providing nursing and
    related primary care services.

2   A neighbourhood nursing service (NNS) should be
    established in each neighbourhood.

3   Each neighbourhood nursing service should be headed
    by a manager chosen for her management skills and
    leadership qualities, and she should be based in the
    neighbourhood.

4   Community midwives, community psychiatric nurses and
    community mental handicap nurses should ensure,
    through their respective managers and the
    neighbourhood nursing manager, that their specialist
    contributions are fully co-ordinated with the work of
    the neighbourhood nursing service.

5   All other specialist nurses who work outside hospital
    should be based in the community and managed as part
    of the neighbourhood nursing service.   Each
    specialist nurse should be assigned to one or more
    neighbourhood services and have the commitment of her
    time to each service specified.

6   The principle should be adopted of introducing the
    nurse practitioner into primary health care.

7   The DHSS should agree a limited list of items and
    simple agents which may be prescribed by nurses as
    part of a nursing care programme, and issue
    guidelines to enable nurses to control drug dosage in
    well-defined circumstances.

8   To establish and be recognised as a primary health
    care team, each general medical practice and the
    community nurses associated with it should come to an
    understanding of the team's objectives and
    individuals' roles within it.

    That understanding should be incorporated into a
    written agreement signed jointly by the practice
    partners and by the manager of the neighbourhood

nursing service on behalf of the relevant health authority.

The agreement should name the doctors and community nurses who together form the primary care team and should guarantee the right of the team members to be consulted on any changes proposed in its composition.

The making of such an agreement should be a qualifying condition for any incentive payments which may be introduced to improve quality in general practice (as suggested in the recent policy statement of the Royal College of General Practitioners).

9   The Government should invite the Health Advisory Service, with its established reputation, credibility and acceptance by the professions, to take on responsibility for identifying and promoting good practice in primary health care.

10 Subsidies to general practitioners enabling them to employ staff to perform nursing duties should be phased out.

11 Within two years the United Kingdom Central Council for Nursing, Midwifery and Health Visiting and the English National Board should introduce a common training course for all first-level nurses wishing to work outside hospital in what are now the fields of health visiting, district nursing and school nursing.

12 The provision of nursing services in the community should remain the responsibility of district health authorities. We would urge, however, that in due course the Government should give consideration to amalgamating family practitioner committees and district health authorities and so bring all primary health care services under the control of one body.

13 A short but thorough manpower planning exercise on a practical (as distinct from purely academic) basis should be undertaken to ensure that the training and supply of community nurses is, and remains at, the appropriate level. The study should be supported by the NHS Management Board as an essential task in reviewing the adequacy and consistency of Regional plans.

14 Health care associations should be formed, each
   covering one or more neighbourhoods.

Part Two

Programme for Action

CONTENTS

TIMESCALE FOR ACTION

If the maximum benefits are to be gained from the recommendations in Part One of the Community Nursing Review report, we believe a rapid programme of implementation is desirable. This will enable improvements to be achieved sooner rather than later and will take advantage of the widespread desire for change.

To assist this process, we propose a challenging timescale for action. The 'start date' will depend on any necessary consultation on the major thrust of the recommendations, but some action may be taken in advance of any national decision. Indeed, many authorities are already working along the lines of some of our suggestions. The suggested timescale therefore quotes the latest schedule for the completion of each of the tasks identified; all times are measured from the date of formal Ministerial endorsement.

For each task a specific 'responsibility' is allocated. In many cases the work will be undertaken by others, for example through delegation, but the actual obligation to achieve the target rests with the named person or bodies.

TIMESCALE FOR ACTION

TIME	RESPONSIBILITY	ACTION
2 months	Health Authority	Agree principles and detailed workplan for district.
3 months		Draw up model agreement for primary health care teams.
6 months		Distribute statements on aims for service to each client group.
6 months	Unit General Manager	Identify neighbourhoods.
9 months		Define neighbourhood nursing services and select managers.
10 months		Run induction courses for neighbourhood nursing managers.
12 months		Formally establish neighbourhood nursing services.
15 months		Complete orientation and team building in each neighbourhood nursing service.
18 months		Reach written agreements with all general practitioners.
12 months	Unit General Manager	Define management information plans.
18 months		Produce basic management information for all neighbourhood nursing services.
2 years	Unit General Manager	Appoint some nurse practitioners in all districts.
1 year	NHS Management Board	Complete practical manpower planning study.
1½ years		Define and introduce management training courses.
1½ years	Secretary of State	Extend Health Advisory Service role to cover all primary health care.
2 years		Introduce legislation for enhanced prescribing rights.
4 years	Secretary of State	Phase out practice nurse subsidy for general practitioners.
4 years		Incorporate 'Primary Health Care Team Agreement' as factor in general practitioner payments.
2 years	UKCC and ENB	Introduce common training for all community nurses.

ACTION PROGRAMME FOR ESTABLISHING NEIGHBOURHOOD NURSING SERVICES

Health authorities, through their general managers, will need to work through the following steps:

IDENTIFYING NEIGHBOURHOODS

1. Objectives and their respective priorities should be clarified for determining the size and boundaries of neighbourhoods, in order, for example, to:

- promote equity of access to services.
- build on existing strengths in the provision of primary care services and to minimise disruption.
- promote co-operation between staff providing different services for the same clients.
- simplify planning the balance of resources across the district.
- maximise the use made of resources available for direct patient care.
- minimise travel, costs and inconvenience for clients and staff.

2. In the light of identified objectives, information should be collated on factors which help define neighbourhoods. These might include:

- pattern of housing, shops and community facilities.
- travelling times between population centres and different parts of the district.
- natural boundaries, such as rivers, roads and railways.
- existing bases for community services provided by health authorities, and catchment areas and caseloads of health visitors, district nurses and midwives.
- school catchment areas.
- the siting of general practitioners' practices and their catchment areas.
- geographical patches of specialist teams.
- census enumeration districts (available from Office of Population Censuses and Surveys) including postal code identifiers for vulnerable groups, such as elderly people, people living alone and people living in poor housing.
- social services administrative divisions and catchment areas of social workers and home helps.

3. Provisional division of the District into neighbourhoods should be made.

4. Consultations on these proposals will need to be carried out with local general practitioners, community nurses, specialist services, local authority social services, education, housing and planning departments, voluntary organisations and consumer groups.

ESTABLISHING NEIGHBOURHOOD NURSING SERVICES

5. When neighbourhood divisions have been agreed, staffing
complements of each proposed neighbourhood nursing service should
be agreed with senior nurse managers. Staffing levels should be
set according to population size weighted for agreed demographic
factors and health, social and environmental indicators.

6. A job description and personal profile for neighbourhood
nursing managers should be drawn up and appointments made. The
clinical role of the nurse managers should also be determined.

7. Appropriate management training should be provided for all
neighbourhood nursing managers, preferably before coming into post
or within six months of the appointment.

8. A timetable should be determined indicating the steps to be
taken in making operational each neighbourhood nursing service.

9. Within that timetable, a training programme should be
established to help managers and nursing staff prepare for the
proposed changes.

10. Arrangements should be made to ensure that all other people
involved, including general practitioners, other health staff,
specialist services, local authority planning, social services,
housing and education departments, voluntary organisations and
consumer groups, are informed of the timetable and the
implications of the changes.

11. A model agreement for primary health care teams should be
drawn up and agreements signed with all general practitioners
willing to enter into the formation of a primary health care team.

12. Links should be established between neighbourhood nursing
services and arrangements agreed for one neighbourhood nursing
service to call on the expertise of a member of another
neighbourhood nursing service, when necessary, for advice on
dealing with a particular problem or meeting a special need.

13. Mechanisms should be determined with other unit managers, as
appropriate, by which neighbourhood nursing services will be able
to obtain the skills and advice of specialist nurses.

14. Clear and effective channels of communication should be
established between senior management and each neighbourhood
nursing manager.

15. The means should be established by which the achievement of
objectives can be monitored.

16. A staff appraisal system should be established relevant to
the new organisational model.

17. The management information required by each neighbourhood nursing service and by senior management should be reviewed and a programme established for achieving it. The cost-effectiveness of existing data collection systems, particularly in relation to the time spent by community nurses in clerical work, should also be considered.

18. Neighbourhood nursing services should be provided with adequate administrative and clerical support and with equipment, such as dictaphones, to ensure that the time spent by nurses on non-nursing duties is reduced to a minimum.

PRIMARY HEALTH CARE TEAM: MODEL AGREEMENT

The manager of the neighbourhood nursing service, on behalf of the district health authority, should aim to reach a joint agreement with each general medical practice in the neighbourhood on the terms on which nursing services will be provided to patients registered with the practice. Such an agreement should be drawn up on the following lines:

1.   The practice shall be able to call on those nurses (named in an annex to the agreement) to provide, or arrange for provision of, nursing services to registered patients, on the understanding that:

a.   Together the practice and the nurses shall constitute a primary health care team.

b.   A written statement of the team's overall aims in providing primary care services to registered patients shall be agreed jointly by the team and be available to patients.

c.   In the light of those aims and information available on the population served, the team shall agree annually a written statement of the team's target objectives for the coming year.

d.   Monthly meetings of the team shall be held to monitor the team's progress in meeting targets and for clinical and other managerial purposes (in accordance with procedures to be agreed jointly).

e.   The means by which referrals shall be made between members of the team and to other agencies shall be agreed jointly by the team in the form of a written protocol.

f.   Each nurse shall take responsibility for acting on referrals from the practice (including referring cases on to other nurses not named in the annex to the agreement) and for reporting back, in whichever way she considers appropriate in the particular circumstances.

g.   The practice and the nurses shall, with the patients' agreement, share records and information.

h.   Patients shall, if they so wish, have direct access to any of the nurses for general health and nursing advice.

j. The nurses shall carry out the whole range of nursing duties deemed necessary to achieve the objectives of the primary health care team, but shall not undertake work outside their professional competence.

k. The practice shall be consulted beforehand on any proposals by the health authority, or its managers, to remove names from, or add names to, the list in the annex to the agreement.

l. The practice shall be consulted on any proposals by the health authority or its managers to limit or extend the role of the nurses as part of the primary health care team.

m. The manager of the neighbourhood nursing service shall be consulted beforehand if and when the practice decides to recruit a new partner.

2. Both parties to the agreement shall provide such information as is available to them on the characteristics of the population served, and on clinical activity and outcomes, in order that they can monitor the performance of the team against its jointly agreed aims and objectives.

3. The agreement shall be reviewed annually by the two parties concerned. Details of the agreement may be renegotiated at any time, given proper notice.

4. The district health authority and the practice shall each have the right to terminate the agreement at three months notice if they so wish.

INTRODUCTION TO CHECK LISTS

The purpose of these checklists is to help achieve improvements in nursing services provided in the community.

The first checklist is to assist health authorities to keep an overall check on the balance of services provided for and in the community. The second is to help managers of neighbourhood nursing services to consider how nurses can work effectively together. The remaining checklists are concerned with improving services for individual client groups.

Underlying many of the points is the concern that nurses need to challenge their traditional roles, work more flexibly and ensure that consistency and co-ordination of care are fostered in order to achieve a more effective and appropriate response to the community's health and nursing needs.

The checklists are for use as working documents, to be referred to regularly, by health authorities and their managers and by nurses, doctors and paramedical staff. They may also be used by other agencies, including community health councils and voluntary organisations, to enable them to assess service provision in their particular area.

It is important that the checklists themselves are reviewed and updated regularly so that service improvement and change continue to be in response to current needs.

CHECKLIST A - FOR HEALTH AUTHORITIES

To monitor and improve the nursing services provided in the community, the following points need to be kept under regular review.

AIMS

A.1   Each health authority should have a written statement of aims, reviewed regularly, for the provision of health care for each client group. These aims should reflect a balance between promoting health, preventing disease and caring for people who are sick, disabled or handicapped. The priorities should be clearly stated. These aims and priorities should then be made available to, and understood by, all staff working in the community.

How is this done?

A.2   The health authority should ensure that services are provided in ways that are sensitive to the differing cultural backgrounds of the population served.

How is this being done?

A.3   Where there is a significant ethnic minority population the health authority should make every effort to recruit and train members from such communities as community nurses.

How is this being done?

RESOURCES

A.4   The balance of resources invested in hospital and the community must be kept under regular review, taking into account the need for resources for health promotion.

How is this being done?

A.5   In reviewing that balance, the health authority should systematically obtain the views and expectations of consumers and give consideration to identified health needs and to the up-take of services.

How is this being done?

A.6   In the allocation of resources to provide services outside
hospitals, the health authority should ensure that local
differences and special needs within the District are recognised.
More resources should be given to localities where health needs
are greatest and to provide for the most vulnerable groups in the
population.

How is this being done?

A.7   If plans are being made to increase the balance of care in
the community, for example, through setting up a hospital-at-home
scheme, increasing the amount of day surgery, promoting earlier
discharge and maintaining more chronically sick, handicapped and
elderly people at home, the corresponding balance of resources
should be transferred from the hospital sector or development
money used to ensure that community services can meet the
increased demands placed on them.

What steps are being taken to ensure this occurs?

A.8   To reduce admission to hospital and to enhance quality of
care, sufficient resources should be invested in the community
services to enable provision of a 24 hour nursing service for all
people requiring such help.

What out-of-hours services are provided?

A.9   The health authority should designate a number of beds as
nursing beds under the management of community nursing staff for
clients who for a short time are in need of more nursing care than
can be given at home.

What steps are being taken to make this provision?

INFORMATION

A.10 The health authority should ensure that information
collected by community nursing staff is appropriate for management
purposes, readily recordable and compatible with financial
information systems for costing purposes.

How is this being done?

A.11 The health authority should ensure that nurses and others
working in the community have ready access to information to give
to the public to help promote individuals' awareness of their
health needs and increase their competence to manage their own
health (for example parent-held child health records; child
development learning packs; individual health care plans;
information on specific handicaps and chronic diseases).

What information is available?

A.12 The health authority should ensure that information is available to the public on all health services provided outside hospital and on how they can influence decisions about service provision and register complaints.

What information is available?

CO-ORDINATION

A.13 The health authority should agree arrangements with local authorities and voluntary agencies to ensure adequate provision of practical domestic help for agreed priority groups.

What are these arrangements?

A.14 The health authority and local authority should be jointly responsible for setting up and maintaining adequate and readily available supplies of aids and equipment for agreed priority groups.

What arrangements exist?

A.15 The health authority should agree with local authorities and voluntary agencies the provision to be made for respite care for different client groups and for supporting informal carers.

What provisions are being made?

A.16 The health authority should recognise the knowledge, expertise and resources of many voluntary organisations and should seek opportunities to work in partnership with them in providing services for particular client groups.

In what ways is the health authority working with voluntary organisations?

A.17 The health authority should have clearly understood links with the family practitioner committee to identify needs in the community and to ensure that health authority staff and family practitioner services work together in the provision of primary health care.

What links exist, and how are the health authority and family practitioner committee working together?

A.18 To encourage a co-ordinated approach to the provision of services in the community, the health authority should ensure that midwifery teams have clear links with the neighbourhood nursing services.

What links exist?

A.19 To encourage a co-ordinated approach to the provision of services in the community, the health authority should ensure that nurses working in the community as part of specialist teams have clear links with the neighbourhood nursing services.

What links exist?

A.20 To avoid fragmentation of care, the health authority should agree on an acceptable balance between provision of services through neighbourhood nursing services and through teams which may be set up to meet the needs of a particular client group for example, a District-wide team for the care of elderly people.

What is the balance between District-wide and neighbourhood nursing service provision?

A.21 There should be clearly understood arrangements between hospital and community nursing staff concerning the admission to hospital and discharge of patients to ensure adequate support is available on their return home.

What are the arrangements?

CHECKLIST B - FOR NEIGHBOURHOOD NURSING MANAGERS

To enable the manager and staff of each neighbourhood nursing service to work together to meet the needs of the locality more effectively, the following points need to be worked through.

IDENTIFICATION OF NEIGHBOURHOOD NEEDS

B.1   The neighbourhood nursing manager, with the nursing staff, should build up a profile of the neighbourhood, covering demographic trends and health, social and environmental characteristics. Sources of information include:

- consumer surveys.
- community health councils.
- age-sex registers held by family practitioner committees.
- data from the health authority on mortality, morbidity and uptake of services, such as immunisation rates, in the particular locality.
- census data covering size and structure of household, standard of housing and social class.
- unemployment rates.
- provision and uptake of other services in the locality, both statutory and voluntary.
- views of general practitioners, social services departments, voluntary organisations and other agencies.

What information is available, and how is it being used?

B.2   The manager and staff should review information available on the current work being undertaken, for example:

- overall and individual workloads.
- number of home visits made to different age groups.
- number of clinic sessions.
- number of people seen in clinics in different age groups.
- client turnover - number of new clients and number of discharges.
- type of nursing work being done.
- dependency levels of clients.
- consumer comments registering satisfaction or complaint.

What is the current work pattern?

B.3 With reference to District policies and comparing the current workload and the neighbourhood profile, the neighbourhood nursing manager should identify needs and suggested priorities for the neighbourhood nursing service.

What are the needs and priorities?

B.4 These needs and priorities should be discussed with general practitioners, specialist nursing and multi-disciplinary teams, local social services departments, voluntary organisations and the community health council.

What arrangements exist for this?

B.5 The manager should be responsible for keeping her senior nurse manager informed about agreed needs and priorities.

What channels of communication exist?

B.6 There should be a clear system for planning action to tackle priorities, setting targets, monitoring the extent to which they are met and reviewing the priorities themselves.

What system exists for this?

CONSUMER ISSUES

B.7 The manager and staff of the neighbourhood nursing service, together with local general practitioners, should agree on methods of publisising the services offered.

How are services publicised?

B.8 The manager and staff of the neighbourhood nursing service, together with local general practitioners, should consider methods of measuring consumer satisfaction with the services offered and involving the public in local service planning.

How is this being done?

B.9 The neighbourhood nursing manager should be an essential member of any local health care association and should make a positive contribution to its success both as a source of information and regarding specific provision.

How is such involvement being pursued?

OPERATIONAL METHODS

B.10 The neighbourhood nursing manager should ensure that members of the neighbourhood nursing service meet regularly, having agreed on the frequency, purpose and structure of the meetings.

When are meetings held and how are they used?

B.11 The manager should keep under review the particular skills, interests and aptitudes of the nurses in the neighbourhood nursing service. The manager should encourage individual staff to develop their particular skills and knowledge further, and should promote new ways of working and greater flexibility of roles. The manager should, in discussion with staff, decide on the best way to deploy the members of the neighbourhood nursing service to meet its priorities.

How is this being done?

B.12 The manager should review the range of tasks undertaken by each skill group and identify ways of maximising the contribution of less skilled staff under the direction of appropriately qualified staff.

How is this being achieved?

B.13 The manager should decide how the work of registered and enrolled nurses and auxiliary staff should be managed in the neighbourhood nursing service.

What are the management arrangements?

B.14 The manager should review the size of the neighbourhood nursing service area, the spread of general practitioners' practices and travelling time, and decide what restrictions, if any, are required on distances travelled by particular staff.

What has been decided?

B.15 The manager, with the nursing staff, should keep under review the balance between home visiting and client contact in the clinic. The balance between working with individual clients and with groups should also be considered.

How is this being done?

B.16 The manager should encourage the members of the neighbourhood nursing service to recognise and make use of each other's particular expertise, and to agree a referral system among themselves.

How is this being done?

B.17 The neighbourhood nursing manager should ensure that group training sessions are made available to foster team working and identification with the neighbourhood served.

What training is available?

RELATIONSHIPS WITH OTHER PROFESSIONALS AND AGENCIES

B.18 The manager should establish links with general practitioner practices in the neighbourhood and seek to reach a signed agreement with each one.

What agreements have been reached with general practitioners?

B.19 The manager, with the nursing staff, should establish and maintain links with other agencies working in the neighbourhood, particularly social services and voluntary organisations. The neighbourhood nursing service should seek to work closely with them, considering for example, ways of working in partnership with voluntary organisations to meet particular client needs and agreeing methods of referral and assessment with social services.

What links exist?

B.20 The manager, with the nursing staff, should establish and maintain links with other health professionals working in the neighbourhood, particularly specialist nurses accountable to other managers, and the paramedical services.

What links exist?

B.21 The neighbourhood nursing manager should ensure that there are clearly understood arrangements for referring clients for specialist help or for obtaining advice or information from a specialist, and for ensuring co-ordination and consistency of care when more than one worker is visiting a particular client or family.

What are these arrangements?

PERSONNEL

B.23 The manager should identify additional training needs of nursing staff and seek to ensure that these are met.

What are these needs, and how are they being met?

B.24 The manager should ensure that professional support is available for the staff and should also promote peer group support.

How is support being provided?

B.25 The manager of the neighbourhood nursing service should be available to advise members on all professional matters. When necessary, the manager should direct the nurse to outside expertise, for example, from the manager of, or expert working in, another neighbourhood nursing service.

How is professional advice made available?

B.26 The manager should monitor the work done by individual nurses to ensure that a high quality of health and nursing care is maintained.

How is this being done?

B.27 The manager, with the nursing staff, should ensure a system is agreed for covering the workload with respect to out-of-hours provision, holidays, study leave and sickness, and should also agree acting-up arrangements in the manager's absence.

What arrangements exist?

CHECKLIST C - MOTHERS-TO-BE AND NEW PARENTS

To monitor and improve nursing and midwifery services provided in the community for mothers-to-be and new parents, the following points need to be kept under regular review.

C.1   Each health authority should have a statement of its broad aims for providing maternity care. These aims should be known and understood by all community midwives, health visitors, other community nursing staff, obstetricians and general practitioners.

How is this being done?

C.2   Every mother and father should have information on, and be able to make, choices about care during the pregnancy, childbirth and postnatal period.

How is this achieved?

C.3   In each District, arrangements should be made between the health authority and family practitioner committee to keep shared care under review. All midwives, obstetricians and general practitioners should understand the arrangements for shared care, how low- and high-risk cases are defined, and the appropriate pattern of care to be provided.

How is this done?

C.4   The policy on home deliveries and 'domino' schemes and the reason for such policies should be made known to parents.

How is this done?

C.5   For the majority of mothers whose pregnancy is considered low risk, antenatal care should be provided primarily by a midwife in association with a general practitioner. An agreed programme of care should be provided which aims to avoid unnecessary duplication of effort between midwives, general practitioners and hospital-based staff.

What arrangements have been agreed?

C.6   The opportunity should be offered to all low risk mothers to have a planned short stay in hospital for the delivery of their baby, leaving normally six hours after the birth. The uptake of such short stay schemes should be kept under review.

What provision is made?

C.7   Each mother needs reliable and consistent advice about her own health care and that of her baby.   To prevent mothers receiving conflicting advice, common policies should be agreed throughout the District, and organisational and management arrangements (for example, small neighbourhood teams operating both in hospital and the community) should be made to minimise the number of midwives and health visitors involved in an individual mother's maternity care.

What arrangements have been made?

C.8   Systematic attempts should be made to find out clients' wishes about parentcraft classes and postnatal support groups, so that the classes and groups provided by health authority staff meet clients' particular needs, and compliment those provided by voluntary organisations.

How is this being done?

C.9   Parents of babies who are in neonatal units need special support both in hospital and at home.

What provision is being made for this?

C.10 Each mother should be offered the opportunity of advice and support from a midwife known to her on a 24-hour basis up to four weeks after the birth of her baby.

What steps are being taken to do this?

C.11 Mothers who choose to take up that offer should not normally be visited at home by a health visitor during that period; support and advice on maternal health and early child care should be provided by the midwife and general practitioner. A system should be agreed locally for determining which mothers should be offered joint care by midwives and health visitors.

What arrangements have been agreed?

C.12 Transfer of care from the midwife to the health visitor should if possible be done in person and promptly at the agreed time.

What provision is there for this?

C.13 All community midwives should have up-to-date knowledge of family planning in order to be able to give appropriate advice.

What arrangements are there for this?

C.14 Midwives, health visitors and general practitioners should be skilled in bereavement counselling.

What provision is there for this?

C.15 In neighbourhoods with significant ethnic minority groups, provision should be made to meet the special needs of mothers-to-be and new parents who come from these communities.

What provision is being made for this?

CHECKLIST D - CHILDREN 0-5 YEARS

To monitor and improve nursing services provided in the community for children from birth to five years old and their parents, the following points need to be kept under regular review.

D.1 Each health authority should have a statement of its broad aims in providing services for children under five years and their parents. All community nurses should be aware of the aims and understand their part in implementing policy.

How is this being done?

D.2 All parents of young children need written information on what health care and advisory services are provided by their family doctor and by health authority staff, and what their purpose and benefits are. The health authority should provide information on its services, together with information on the skills of the different staff available.

How is this being done?

D.3 Parents should be given consistency of advice and services offered. Common policies should be agreed throughout the District on such child care matters as infant feeding, and all health professionals should be encouraged to follow them. The ages at which developmental screening and immunisation schedules are carried out should be agreed in each District between the general practitioners, clinical medical officers and community nurses.

What provision is being made for this?

D.4 New parents need to be able to have advice on child care and child health matters on a 24-hour basis during their child's first months. Each health authority should ensure that this is available and that staff who run such a service are adequately trained to be able to give advice, over the telephone, if necessary.

What provision is being made?

D.5 To avoid duplication of advice to new parents, a system should be agreed locally for determining which categories of parents should be offered joint care by midwives and health visitors in the postnatal period, and for determining when the midwife and the health visitor both need to visit the home.

What system has been agreed?

D.6 New parents need information on how their child is likely to develop as well as information on what they can do to enhance the good development of the child physically, emotionally, intellectually and socially. A child development learning pack should be available for new parents.

What provision is there for this?

D.7 All health care staff should aim to promote parents' confidence and competence in their parenting abilities. For new parents this may be achieved by providing, on a partnership basis, a structured programme of support and information on how best to develop these skills (for example, the Bristol Child Development Project).

What steps are being taken to achieve this?

D.8 As parents' confidence and competence grow, the need for home visiting lessens, and advice and support can become more clinic- or centre-based. Home visiting will still be of value to some groups of parents. A system for determining priority of need for home visiting by community nursing staff should be developed and visits made by appointment whenever possible.

What provision is there for this?

D.9 Parents of children who have a handicap will need specialist advice. This advice needs to be readily accessible and in keeping with current research and thinking. A resource centre for such parents in the locality should be available where parents may gain advice and support from both the statutory and voluntary services.

What provision is being made?

D.10 Parents of children who have a handicap need regular guidance and support from a community nurse who is adequately prepared for such a role.

What arrangements are made for this?

D.11 Voluntary organisations can provide an excellent resource for parents who have children with a handicap. Community nurses should know the range of organisations and their brief. Community nurses should have access to a directory of services, both statutory and voluntary, which will be of use to parents of children who have a handicap.

What provision is there for this?

D.12 Children whose parents or carers are unable for whatever reason, to cope with their responsibilities as parents need the assurance that other agencies will be involved on their behalf as and when the need arises. Community nurses need to know how and when to involve such services.

What provision is there for this?

D.13 Each health authority should have written indicators for community nursing staff to use to highlight which children may be at risk of developmental delay, sudden infant death, neglect or abuse. These indicators should be agreed with clinical medical officers, general practitioners and paediatricians and be adhered to throughout the District.

What steps are being taken to achieve this?

D.14 All community nurses working with young children, including those working in health centre treatment rooms, should be aware of the signs and symptoms of child abuse and know what action to take in accordance with local policies.

What provision is being made for this?

D.15 In the case of suspected or actual child abuse, arrangements should be made for a health visitor experienced in this field to work jointly with the family's regular health visitor if the latter has insufficient experience.

What arrangements are made for this?

D.16 Community nurses working with families where child abuse is suspected or has occurred should have close monitoring and supervision by their nurse manager.

What provision is there for this?

D.17 Children who are ill should be nursed at home, admission to hospital being avoided whenever possible. If a child is admitted to hospital the community nurse should be involved before discharge and draw up, with the parents and hospital staff, a care plan for the child.

What provision is there for this?

D.18 When sick children are nursed at home, unless specialist nursing skills are required, all care and support should normally be provided by the family's regular community nurse. Unnecessary duplication of effort by neighbourhood nursing staff should be avoided.

How is this being done?

D.19 When parents and community nurses need the extra support and skills of trained paediatric nurses, these nurses should normally guide the regular nurses but in some cases they may need to be involved in direct care.

What provision is made?

D.20 In the case of all children with special needs (for example, children who are sick or handicapped or at risk of neglect or abuse) arrangements should be made that when more than one professional is involved with a family, advice and care provided by community nurses is co-ordinated locally with other agencies concerned.

What arrangements are being made for this?

D.21 In neighbourhoods with significant ethnic minority groups, community nurses should work with individuals and groups who can highlight these groups' particular health needs. Consideration should be given to the employment and training, as a short-term measure, of workers from the community who can advise people from ethnic minority groups (particularly people new to the country) on health matters and on how to use health services.

What provision is there for this?

D.22 In such neighbourhoods, interpreters for the health professionals should be trained in interpreting skills and the community nurses should be trained in how to make use of their skills. The interpreters should also have a role in acting on behalf of the consumer to ensure that the service delivered is sensitive to the health needs and culture of particular groups.

What provision is there for this?

D.23 All services offered by community nurses should be viewed as a partnership with the parents and the child. Parental access to records kept and to meetings involving their welfare and that of their children will enhance the status of this partnership.

What is being done to achieve this?

D.24 Systematic attempts should be made to find out parents' wishes about the provision of home and clinic-based services and whether current provision reflects those wishes.

How is this done?

CHECKLIST E - CHILDREN 5-16 YEARS

To monitor and improve nursing services provided in the community for children aged from five to 16 years, the following points need to be kept under regular review.

E.1   Each health authority should have a statement of its broad aims for providing services for schoolchildren and their parents. These aims should be agreed annually with the education authorities and should be known and understood by community nurses, clinical medical officers, general practitioners, teaching staff and the education welfare service.

How is this being done?

E.2   Each school should have a named nurse and a named doctor who are able to work together to objectives agreed with the school. These objectives should be reviewed annually.

How is this being achieved?

E.3   In order to gain full benefit from their educational experience, children need to be in their optimum state of health. Parents and teachers need to be aware of what might hinder this. They need information about the normal development of the child and why certain defects may affect learning ability.

What provision is made for this?

E.4   Parents need to be able to make informed choices about how the health care needs of their child are met during his school years. Decisions about a child's health and related educational needs should be made by parents in partnership with health and educational staff.

How is this being done?

E.5   Children, parents and teachers need to know the role and skills of the school nurse. Children should be able to have access to the school nurse in confidence on any health-related matter.

How is this being achieved?

E.6   The nurse's skills in health surveillance and in providing
health advice for this age group should be regularly updated. She
should also have opportunities to use and develop her skills in
different settings inside and outside of school with parents as
well as children.

What provision is there for this?

E.7   Procedures for screening all children in schools for
particular health or developmental problems should be undertaken
only when this is proven to be cost-effective. The need for
screening should be kept under review.

How is this being done?

E.8   Every school nurse should understand the procedures under
the 1981 Education Act through which needs for special educational
provision are identified.

How is this being achieved?

E.9   All community nurses working with children of school age
should have access to expert advice on educational and
developmental health matters. They should be able to seek advice
from experienced nurses in the field not necessarily based in
their neighbourhood nursing service.

How is this being done?

E.10 Children who have handicap and their parents may need
particular support from the school nurse. The nurse should have
the skills to deal with the physical and psychological needs of
the child and know when and how to involve other specialist
workers who may share in the care of the child.

What provision is being made for this?

E.11 All community nurses working with this age group should have
the knowledge and skills to detect signs of physical, emotional
and sexual abuse.

How are their knowledge and skills kept up-to-date?

E.12 Every school nurse should understand how and when to inform
her nursing, clinical medical officer and general practitioner
colleagues of individual and group health needs as they arise.
This should be done as far as possible with the child's and
parent's consent.

What arrangements are there for this?

E.13 Close links should be maintained between community nurses working with this age group, teachers and the local health education department for identifying current health education needs of schoolchildren and planning how best to meet them.

How is this being achieved?

E.14 Community nurses working with this age group should establish links with education welfare officers, child guidance staff, parent-teacher associations and other relevant agencies in the neighbourhood.

What steps are being taken to achieve this?

CHECKLIST F - ADOLESCENTS AND YOUNG ADULTS

To monitor and improve nursing services provided in the community for adolescents and young adults, the following points need to be kept under regular review.

F.1 Each health authority should have a statement of its broad aims for providing services for adolescents and young adults. All community nurses should be aware of the aims and understand their part in implementing policy.

How is this being done?

F.2 Young people need information on how life-styles and behaviour can affect their health, how to look after themselves, and where to get professional advice on health matters.

What information is available locally and how is it disseminated?

F.3 Health care professionals need to recognize that young people have different perceptions of their health needs and of the effects of their life-styles from those of their parents and older generations. Specific training and other help should be provided for those community nurses who work regularly with young adults and adolescents.

What provision is being made?

F.4 Health advice for young people should be offered as part of the primary care services available for the local community, but in ways that will avoid stigma to those who seek help.

What special efforts are made to encourage young people to use primary care services?

F.5 Young people need also to be assured that any health problems they have will not be discussed by their doctor or nurse with their parents, partners or others, unless they agree.

How is this done?

F.6 Young people who are unwilling, for whatever reason, to seek advice from their family doctor should be able to have direct access to an appropriately trained community nurse.

What arrangements exist?

F.7   In each neighbourhood, consideration should be given by general practitioners and the neighbourhood nursing service to advisory centres that might be provided for young people, and where they should be sited, (for example, drop-in clinics on matters such as drug abuse, alcohol problems, sexually transmitted diseases, family planning, preparing for pregnancy and parenthood, sexual identity).

What provision is being made?

F.8   Parents need access to advice on the types of health problems that might arise with this age group.

What provision is there for this?

F.9   Close links should be maintained between neighbourhood nursing services and the local health education department so that the health needs of adolescents can be kept under regular review.

How is this arranged?

CHECKLIST G - WELL ADULTS

To monitor and improve nursing services provided in the community for well adults, the following points need to be kept under regular review.

G.1   Each health authority should have a statement of its broad aims for the promotion of health in well adults. All community nurses should be aware of the aims and understand their part in implementing policy.

How is this being done?

G.2   Every opportunity should be taken by health care staff to encourage adults to take an interest in, and responsibility for, their own health. Information should be available on all aspects of health promotion so that their competence to manage their own health is increased.

What information is available?

G.3   Advisory, screening and health promotion services provided by community nurses for example, well men's and well women's clinics, should be well publicised and provided at times and in places convenient for local people. Consideration should be given to evening or Saturday morning clinics and to clinic sessions in work-places or community centres.

What provision is being made?

G.4   In response to local need consideration should be given to setting up groups and encouraging self-help groups for example, groups for smokers or informal carers.

What steps are being taken to identify and meet these needs?

G.5   Particular consideration should be given to people in the pre-retirement age group to prepare them for a healthier retirement and old age. Group health education sessions could be held or a full health check offered and individual health care plans drawn up and held by the clients.

What provision is being made for this age group?

G.6 Some adults may be particularly vulnerable to health problems or may not make full use of health services for example, homeless people or those who are not registered with a general practitioner. Efforts should be made to identify these groups and opportunities taken to encourage and facilitate a greater interest in health care.

What is being done?

G.7 Health education and health promotion services should be provided in ways which are sensitive to, and accepting of, individual and group differences such as those of age, culture and life-style.

How is this being done?

G.8 The training needs of nurses working with well adults should be reviewed and in-service training provided with particular regard to developing group work skills.

What in-service training is available?

G.9 Services provided by nurses should be co-ordinated with services provided by other health professionals and other statutory and voluntary agencies in the locality.

How is this being done?

CHECKLIST H - ACUTELY ILL AND TERMINALLY ILL PEOPLE

To monitor and improve nursing services provided in the community for acutely ill or terminally ill people, the following points need to be kept under regular review.

H.1   Each health authority should have a statement of its broad aims for providing services for acutely ill and terminally ill people.   All community nurses should be aware of the aims and understand their part in implementing policy.

How is this being done?

H.2   Acutely and terminally ill people who are nursed at home are likely to come into contact with a varied number of health and welfare professionals.   All professionals should follow a team approach and individual care plans should be drawn up which are agreed and understood by the patient and any carers involved.

What steps are being taken to see that this is done?

H.3   Nursing care and support may be required over a 24 hour period.

What provision is made for this?

H.4   Some patients need specialist services such as teams involved with pain control and paramedical services. There should be an updated directory of these services available for general practitioners and community nurses.

What steps are being taken to achieve this?

H.5   Where specialist teams, such as those who work with terminally ill people, are involved, they must work closely with the general practitioners and community nurses to effect optimum support for patients and carers. Specialist teams, the general practitioners and community nurses should understand each other's roles.

What steps are being taken to achieve this?

H.6   Specialist teams should be available for consultation by community nurses on clients other than those with whom they are currently involved.

How is this done?

H.7 The needs of carers in these situations need to be adequately assessed. Nurses can best assess the practical and emotional needs if, as part of their in-service training, they spend time in place of, or working alongside, the carer.

What steps are being taken to achieve this?

H.8 Each health authority should ensure jointly with the local authority social services department and voluntary organisations that individual carers' needs are assessed and met, and that the type and level of practical help and respite care facilities provided locally are adequate.

What arrangements are being made for this?

H.9 Patients and carers need access to information, particularly on welfare benefits, home aids and equipment, and other voluntary and statutory services, so that they can make informed choices. Community nurses should keep regularly updated on this information and should know the criteria used by local authority staff for the provision of the home-help service and equipment so that assessments are not duplicated.

What provision is being made for this?

H.10 A laundry service, as well as a supply of extra linen, is often required for these patients.

What provision is there for this?

H.11 Some people may benefit from having a volunteer stay with them for periods or visit them regularly each day because they live alone or cannot depend on such care from a relative. This may involve a joint arrangement with the local authority social services department and voluntary organisations.

What provision is made for this?

H.12 Good practice in nursing acutely ill and terminally ill people must be maintained and nurses should have the opportunity to develop their skills through in-service training and have their work regularly monitored. The acquisition of skills in bereavement counselling will be important for those working with terminally ill people.

What steps are being taken to do this?

H.13 It is important that patients and their carers feel able to discuss and review the service and nursing care they are being offered. To be able to do this they need to know whom to approach on such matters.

What provision is there for this?

H.14 Voluntary organisations are a useful source of information and support for these groups. Formal links should be made by the health authority. They should be involved in the planning of new services related to their field, and community nurses should have good information on their role and skills.

What steps are being taken to achieve this?

H.15 Community nurses with most experience of these groups of patients can have much to contribute to discussions on how to achieve the best care possible. They should be involved when services are reviewed by health authorities.

How is this done?

CHECKLIST J - PEOPLE WHO ARE CHRONICALLY SICK OR PHYSICALLY DISABLED

To monitor and improve nursing services provided in the community for people who are chronically sick or physically disabled, the following points need to be kept under regular review.

J.1   Each health authority should have a statement of its broad aims for providing services for people who are chronically sick and physically disabled. All community nurses should be aware of the aims and understand their part in implementing policy.

How is this being done?

J.2   People who are chronically sick or physically disabled need serivces that will enable them to live independently in their own homes and to enjoy a good quality of life. Professionals should work in partnership with clients and their carers in such a way that independence is fostered.

How is this approach put into practice?

J.3   All clients and their carers should know how to contact a suitably experienced nurse for advice or information.

What provision is there for this?

J.4   Clients who are coping independently should have the opportunity to be visited regularly by a nurse for advice, support, health education and the early detection of problems.

What visiting schemes exist?

J.5   When home nursing care is required, care plans should be drawn up and maintained with the agreement and understanding of the client and his family or carers.

How are clients and carers involved in the use of care plans?

J.6   Nursing care should, whenever possible, be provided to suit the convenience of clients. For example, help for people getting up and going to bed should be provided in the early morning and at the end of the evening.

How is the acceptability of services kept under review?

J.7   It is important that clients and carers are able to discuss and review the service and nursing care they are being offered and to request a change of nurse if necessary. To do this, they need to know whom to approach on such matters.

What provision is there for this?

J.8 Nurses working with people who are chronically sick or physically disabled should be aware not only of the health but of the domestic, social and economic needs of this client group, as these may be of more significance than the illness or handicap itself. They should be able to advise on how clients may get support from other agencies.

What steps are taken to ensure that all these needs are considered?

J.9   All primary health care workers should understand the role of specialist nurses providing advice and support to meet particular health needs and know how and when to make referrals or seek specialist advice. While specialists will sometimes work directly with the client, they should also be a resource to other nurses and pass on their skills to them.

How are specialist nursing services used?

J.10 The services provided by physiotherapists, occupational therapists, speech therapists, chiropodists and dieticians are of particular importance to people who are chronically sick or physically disabled.   There should be clearly understood arrangements for referring clients to these services. Nurses should work closely with the paramedical staff and take opportunities to learn from them.

What arrangements exist?

J.11 When more than one agency or health care professional is involved with a client, it is particularly important to ensure that care is co-ordinated and consistent. The designation of a key worker should be considered.

What arrangements exist?

J.12 Informal carers need services which include practical help, respite care, advice on their own health, teaching on how to look after the client, and psychological support.

What services are available?

J.13 There should be joint working and partnership schemes with other agencies in the locality, particularly social services and voluntary organisations, to ensure that services are co-ordinated and that the available resources are being used to the best advantage.

What arrangements exist for this?

CHECKLIST K - PEOPLE WITH MENTAL HEALTH PROBLEMS

To monitor and improve nursing services provided in the community for people with mental health problems, the following points need to be kept under regular review.

K.1   Each health authority should have a statement of its broad aims for providing services for people with mental health problems. All community nurses should be aware of the aims and understand their part in implementing policy.

How is this being done?

K.2   Health services provided in the community for people with mental health problems should build on the resources already available in each neighbourhood and reflect the particular needs and wishes of the local population. Local resources could, for example, provide befriending schemes.

What mechanisms exist to do this?

K.3   Facilities should be provided in the community to help raise the level of functioning of individuals with mental health problems. These facilities should include work-related schemes, drop-in centres and aids to daily living and social skills training schemes.

What facilities exist?

K.4   The care of people in the community with chronic or severe mental disorders should be the primary concern of specialist multi-disciplinary teams in collaboration with general practitioners. Each team would usually comprise psychiatrists, psychologists, psychiatric nurses, occupational therapists and social workers.

What arrangements exist?

K.5   All primary health care workers in regular contact with people with mental health problems should understand the role of the specialist multi-disciplinary team and know how and when to make referrals or seek expert advice.

How is this done?

K.6 Community psychiatric nurses should normally be members of the specialist team but be able to work closely with neighbourhood nursing services and primary health care teams. When a client or his family requires both specialist help and general primary health care, a mechanism should be agreed (for example, a key worker) to co-ordinate care and to prevent undesirable duplication of effort.

What arrangements exist?

K.7 Individual care plans should be drawn up, which are agreed and understood by the client and all workers involved. These care plans must be reviewed regularly so that the care and treatment given continue to be appropriate to the clients' needs.

How are care plans developed and used?

K.8 Information, support including day-time relief, and training, when appropriate, should be provided for the informal carers of people suffering from chronic mental illness.

What support and training programmes exist?

K.9 Clients and their carers should have easy access to information, help and advice on a 24-hour basis within the community from a specialist in mental health.

What provision exists for this?

K.10 Training should be provided for primary care workers in the early detection and management of mental health problems, including postnatal depression and child behavioural problems.

How is this being done?

K.11 Primary care workers should be able to call on specialist teams for expert advice, when appropriate, in dealing with problems such as violence, drug and alcohol misuse, breakdown in family functioning and the effects of unemployment.

What expert advice is available?

K.12 A system should be established for identifying and monitoring the progress of people who live in temporary, emergency or unregistered residential accommodation who because of their psychiatric problems require continuous or intermittent care and treatment.

How is this being achieved?

K.13 In neighbourhoods with significant ethnic minority groups, provision should be made to meet the special needs of people with mental health problems and their families who come from these communities.

What provision is being made for this?

CHECKLIST L - PEOPLE WITH A MENTAL HANDICAP

To monitor and improve services provided in the community for people with a mental handicap, the following points need to be kept under regular review.

L.1   Each health authority should have a statement of its broad aims for providing services for people with a mental handicap. All community nurses should be aware of the aims and understand their part in implementing policy.

How is this being done?

L.2   The services provided in the community for people with a mental handicap should build on the resources already available in each neighbourhood and reflect the particular needs and wishes of the local population.

What mechanisms exist to do this?

L.3   Each person with a mental handicap should have the opportunity to participate in a purposeful programme of daily activities, to develop relationships and participate in local community life.

How is this being encouraged?

L.4   Each health authority should have one or more specialist teams for people with a mental handicap which are able to integrate the work of statutory and voluntary agencies locally.

What arrangements exist?

L.5   A prime responsibility of specialist teams should be the identification of the needs of people with a mental handicap and the drawing up of individual programme plans, which are reviewed regularly, to enable them to develop their full potential. For each client, a key worker should be designated in the team to co-ordinate care and to act as the person's advocate.

How is this being done?

L.6   The normal health care needs of a person with a mental handicap should be met by his general practitioner and community nurse. Each primary health care team should determine how to facilitate access to primary care services by clients registered with them who have a mental handicap.

How is this being done?

L.7   All primary health care workers should understand the role
of the specialist team and know how and when to refer clients to
them and to seek advice.

How is this done?

L.8   Primary care and specialist teams working in the same
neighbourhoods should foster links to ensure a more co-ordinated
approach to the planning and delivery of services.

What links exist?

L.9   Informal carers of a person with a mental handicap
particulary need teaching on how to help him to become more self-
reliant and to fulfil his potential.

How is this need catered for?

L.10 Arrangements should be made for respite care for informal
carers, and opportunities provided for the person with a mental
handicap to have breaks away from home which may also serve as a
preparation for independent living.

What provision is made?

L.11 In neighbourhoods with significant ethnic minority groups,
provision should be made to meet the special needs of people with
a mental handicap and their families who come from these
communities.

What provision is being made for this?

CHECKLIST M - ELDERLY PEOPLE

To monitor and improve nursing services provided in the community for elderly people, the following points need to be kept under regular review.

M.1 Each health authority should have a statement of its broad aims for providing services for elderly people. All community nurses should be aware of the aims and understand their part in implementing policy.

How is this being done?

M.2 Elderly people need relevant health information and advice so that good health can be encouraged and their competence to manage their own health increased.

How is this need being met?

M.3 Primary care services should provide programmes for the early detection of disease or disability in elderly people.

What is being provided?

M.4 As part of such programmes elderly people who have particular problems concerning health or daily living, or those considered at risk for any reason, for example those living alone, those over 85 years of age or the recently bereaved should be identified and followed up by regular and frequent home visiting.

How is this being done?

M.5 For those elderly people requiring home nursing care, individual care plans should be drawn up and maintained, with the agreement and understanding of patients and their carers.

How are patients and carers involved in the use of care plans?

M.6 Sufficient care including, when necessary, intensive support from community staff and a 24-hour nursing service, should be available to allow sick, frail or disabled elderly people to remain at home and to prevent unnecessary hospital admission.

What provision is available?

M.7   Each neighbourhood nursing service should have a system for determining priorities of need for home nursing care for elderly people.

How are priorities determined?

M.8   All nurses working with elderly people should be able to give advice on how their clients may obtain other services such as paramedical services, aids, equipment, domestic support and welfare benefits.

What steps are taken to ensure that this is done?

M.9   Each health authority should ensure that specialist advice and support are available to meet the needs of elderly people who undergo mood, behaviour or personality changes or have memory deficits.   All nurses working with elderly people should understand how they can obtain this specialist help for clients or their carers.

What provision is made?

M.10 For elderly people with problems relating to continence, specialist advice and teaching should be available, with the emphasis on promoting continence and so helping to maintain the independence of the client.

What specialist provision is available?

M.11 When more than one agency or health care professional is involved in the care of an elderly person arrangements should exist to ensure that care is co-ordinated and advice is consistent. The appointment of a key worker should be considered.

What arrangements exist?

M.12 When an elderly person is admitted to hospital, consideration should be given to his home situation and the home care services that he will need so that arrangements can be made for an early and successful return home.

How is this done?

M.13 All health care professionals should work in partnership with the informal carers of elderly people, helping them to determine what services they may need, including practical help, respite care, day or night sitting, advice on their own health, teaching on how to look after the elderly person, and psychological support.

What provision is made for these various needs?

M.14 It is important that clients and carers are able to discuss and review the services and nursing care thay are being offered and to request changes. To do this, they need to know whom to approach on such matters.

What provision is there for this?

M.15 There should be written guidelines for the identification of elderly people who may be at risk of or subject to physical or emotional abuse, and on the action to be taken. Community nurses should be aware of these guidelines and be able to take appropriate action.

What guidelines are available?

M.16 Each local authority elderly person's home should have a named nurse from the neighbourhood nursing service for advice and professional support.

What provision is made for this?

M.17 Nursing services provided for elderly people in each neighbourhood should be co-ordinated with those of other health professionals, voluntary organsiations, local authority departments and other relevant agencies to enusre that resources are being used in the best way to meet needs.

What arrangements exist for this?

Printed in the UK for HMSO by Hobbs the Printers of Southampton
(2060/86) Dd739956 C50 8/86 G3379